Family-Based Palliative Care

Family-Based Palliative Care

Family-Based Palliative Care

Jane Marie Kirschling
Editor

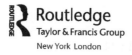

Routledge
Taylor & Francis Group
New York London

First published 1990 by The Haworth Press, Inc.

Published 2017 by Routledge
711 Third Avenue, New York, NY 10017, USA
2 Park Square, Milton Park, Abingdon, Oxon OX14 4RN

First issued in paperback 2018

Routledge is an imprint of the Taylor & Francis Group, an informa business

Family-Based Palliative Care has also been published as *The Hospice Journal*, Volume 6, Number 2 1990.

Library of Congress Cataloging-in-Publication Data

Family-based palliative care / Jane Marie Kirschling, editor.
    p. cm.
    "Has also been published as The hospice journal, volume 6, number 2 1990" – T.p. verso.
    Includes bibliographical references.
    ISBN 1-56024-039-3 (alk. paper)
    1. Terminal care. 2. Hospice care. 3. Terminally ill – Family relationships. I. Kirschling, Jane Marie.
R726.8.F35   1990
362.1'75 – dc20   90-39008
                                                CIP

ISBN 13: 978-1-138-99095-1 (pbk)
ISBN 13: 978-1-56024-039-6 (hbk)

Family-Based Palliative Care

CONTENTS

ABOUT THE EDITOR

Jane Marie Kirschling, RN, DNS, is on the faculty at the Oregon Health Sciences University in the Department of Family Nursing. The focus of her research and clinical practice has been on issues related to death and dying and family caregiving for the terminally ill older persons. During the past 10 years, she has worked with hospice programs in Indiana and Oregon. She received her Baccalaureate in Nursing from Viterbo College and her Masters and Doctoral degrees in Psychiatric/Mental Health Nursing from Indiana University.

Family-Based Palliative Care

Family-Based Palliative Care

Preface

Increasingly families confronted with the terminal illness and eventual death of one of its members have the option to receive hospice care. Unlike traditional health care where the individual is typically the client, the family is viewed as the unit of care by hospice providers with holistic care being emphasized.

This special volume presents theory, practice, and research related to family based care. The volume begins with a conceptual framework for working with hospice families as clients. Clinical examples from hospice are used to illustrate the application of the framework in practice. Next, two qualitative studies, one conducted in a Northeastern city in the United States and one conducted in Western Canada, are presented. The study conducted in the United States describes the sources of stress for caregiving families enrolled in an oncology hospice program. The Canadian study describes the work of patients who have advanced cancer and their spouses while they remain in their home environment.

The fourth article describes the results of a methodological study that was undertaken with family members caring for a terminally ill older person in the Pacific Northwest. Both positive and negative dimensions of social support were explored with family caregivers receiving hospice care. The final article reports on a case study from a hospice program in the Southwest. The case study technique was used to describe and evaluate the staff's efforts in providing family based care.

As the editor of this volume I would like to express my appreciation to the many professional people who reviewed manuscripts. Their willingness to share their expertise and thoughtful review was invaluable to me. I would also like to thank all of the persons who contributed manuscripts for consideration; it is their efforts that made this special volume become a reality. Finally, I would like to thank David Dush. I appreciate the opportunity to work on this volume and his support during the process.

It is hoped that this collection of papers will stimulate hospice care providers to reflect on their own experiences in caring for families. It is also hoped that hospice programs will continue to participate in research activities and theory development related to family based care.

Jane Marie Kirschling
Oregon Health Sciences University
Dept. of Family Nursing

A Conceptual Framework for Caring for Families of Hospice Patients

Joanne E. Hall
Jane Marie Kirschling

SUMMARY. Hospice caregivers are usually family-focused in their practice with individual clients. Less often is the entire family as a unit considered the client. The authors present a conceptual framework for working with hospice families as clients. Their perspective incorporates concepts of the family as a system, the family life cycle, and the components of professional practice. Clinical examples illustrate the application of the framework in practice.

The hospice movement has long been associated with family-focused care. The family frequently is viewed as the context in which the hospice patient lives and as the group of people most personally concerned with the patient's care. What sometimes has been less explicit is a view of the family as a system which in itself may be considered the client. This article presents a conceptual framework that was derived from a synthesis of concepts drawn from general systems, family development, crisis, role, and communication theory. The purpose of this article is to increase hospice

Joanne E. Hall, RN, PhD, has worked clinically with families experiencing developmental and situational crises and taught family theory for more than 25 years. Her current research is focused on family healing and family peacemaking, particularly between middlescent adults and their aging parents. Dr. Hall is Professor of Nursing at the Oregon Health Sciences University, Department of Mental Health Nursing, 3181 SW Sam Jackson Park Road, Portland, OR 97201. Jane Marie Kirschling, RN, DNS, has worked clinically with families receiving hospice care in Indiana and Oregon since 1982. Her current research is focused on the experiences of family caregivers for terminally ill elderly, both prior to, and after the death of their relative. Dr. Kirschling is Associate Professor of Nursing, Oregon Health Sciences University.

1

team members' understanding of the family as a client, enabling them to interact with families in ways that promote family functioning when a family member is dying.

The article is organized according to four major areas. The first area is a brief description of conceptual frameworks in general. The second major area is the family as a system. Family life cycle is the third area. The last area is components of practice. Three case examples from the second author's clinical practice are used to illustrate how theory and practice interface.

CONCEPTUAL BASIS
FOR UNDERSTANDING THE FAMILY AS CLIENT

Conceptual Framework

A conceptual framework is a perspective for viewing the world, composed of a set of related concepts which function as a frame of reference to help people make sense out of their experience. The advantage of a conceptual framework is that it sensitizes professional caregivers to aspects of the family which are significant in caring for the hospice patient. On the other hand, it also can desensitize caregivers to aspects of the family that are unrelated to the concepts in their framework. A conceptual framework of the family should not be confused with an actual family which may possess characteristics very different from those emphasized by an abstract, symbolic representation of the family as a system. Once these limitations are recognized, caregivers will find a conceptual framework useful in their work with families.

The conceptual framework presented here combines a general systems perspective with knowledge of family development and the components of practice commonly used by helping professionals regardless of their discipline. In Figure 1, a cube is used to represent the interaction among these three sets of related concepts. Family as a system, family life cycle, and components of practice form the three dimensions of the model. These dimensions can serve as a way of thinking about families in general as well as a guide for the assessment and planning interventions with specific families.

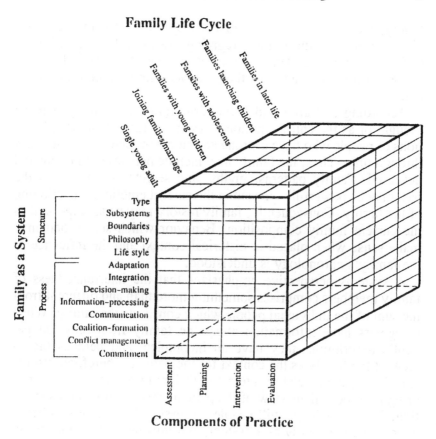

Family Life Cycle

Families in later life
Families launching children
Families with adolescents
Families with young children
Joining families/marriage
Single young adult

Family as a System

Structure
- Type
- Subsystems
- Boundaries
- Philosophy
- Life style

Process
- Adaptation
- Integration
- Decision-making
- Information-processing
- Communication
- Coalition-formation
- Conflict management
- Commitment

Assessment · Planning · Intervention · Evaluation

Components of Practice

Figure 1. Conceptual framework for working with families.

The Family as a System

Definition of Family

Theorists disagree about what constitutes a family (Burgess & Locke, 1953; Carter & McGoldrick, 1988; McCormack, 1974; Terkelson, 1980). It is our belief that arguments about definition are beside the point. If people say they are a family, then they are a family, regardless of whether or not they are related by marriage, birth and/or adoption. In the caregiving situation, the self-definition of family is the important one for it determines how the individuals relate to each other and how they interact with hospice team members.

According to Carter and McGoldrick (1988), a family may be thought of as the entire emotional system of three or more generations of people who have a strong emotional involvement that exists through time. Thus, the family may include persons both living and deceased. Family patterns, myths, and secrets originating in the past may be powerfully present in the current emotional functioning of the family. Consequently, family history may be as important as the current family composition. Behavior which seems odd may make sense when placed in historical context and the influence of the family's chronology is understood.

A systems perspective emphasizes that the interrelatedness of family members comprises something more than and different from the sum of the individual people which constitute the family. When caregivers have information about the family from only the patient's description, they have an incomplete and perhaps biased view of the family as the context for the patient. Therefore, professional caregivers need to interact with family members in order to bring into focus their view of the patient, their family and its situation. This knowledge will enable professional caregivers to better understand the family as a system, and thus be able to minister to the family as a whole as well as to the patient as an individual.

Philosophy of Family Care

A systems perspective is compatible with a philosophy which considers human beings to be persons of worth regardless of their circumstances, who are capable of self-reflection and making their own decisions. Individuals are believed to have the capacity to relate creatively in families in order to support and care for each other. Families are viewed as interrelated, interdependent, interacting complex organisms, constantly influencing and being influenced by their environment. Families are open systems. This openness makes it possible for hospice caregivers to make a difference in the quality of the family's and the client's life at a crucial time in their history. A general systems orientation nurtures a hopeful philosophy of caregiving which recognizes change, learning and growth as possible (Sills & Hall, 1985). Individuals and families do change, sometimes quite unexpectedly and positively, at crisis times.

Family Structure

In addition to nurturing a hopeful philosophy for hospice care, a general systems perspective offers a way to collect and organize data for family assessment which in turn guides intervention with clients and families. As seen in Figure 1, families possess components of both structure and process which serve as the locus of family strengths and/or limitations or dysfunctions.

Family structure refers to the static arrangement of the family's parts at a given moment in time (Bertrand, 1972). It includes the characteristics of the family which make it recognizable as a system and mark it as a separate entity. When viewed through time, family structure appears to change very slowly; yet when these changes do occur, they are in the nature of a sudden leap from one structural form to another. These changes are associated with predictable family transitions, such as the anticipated death of an aging family member. Changes in family structure which occur off schedule usually are very disruptive, as when the family experiences the death of a child. Anticipated or not, death is always disruptive to families. Therefore, hospice team members come in contact with families at a time when they are anticipating a profound structural change. Important components of family structure to be considered when working with these families are shown in Figure 1 and include the family type, subsystems, boundaries, philosophy, and lifestyle.

Type. Families can be typed in a number of ways. For instance, socio-economic class and ethnic background are factors which categorize families and which many health care providers consider when planning patient care. Less often considered are membership arrangement and transactional modes.

Terms describing the membership arrangement include nuclear, extended, multigenerational, single-parent, childless, and blended families. Family-of-origin, family of procreation, adoptive family, and foster family are additional ways of categorizing family structure. What one knows in general about a membership arrangement gives rise to clinical hunches about the nature of a particular family which then need to be confirmed or disqualified through further family assessment.

Prevailing transactional mode refers to the customary way the family members interact with each other and the family interacts with its environment. Members may conduct the business of being a family in any of the following manners: Gemeinschaft, team-cooperative, legal-bureaucratic, bargaining, and coercion (Bredemeier, n.d.). Gemeinschaft refers to a type of family that is exemplified by relationships in which solidarity, loyalty, and care prevails. The members are committed to each other, sentiments run high, and mutual caring and concern dominates. In times of crisis, mutual support may help to mitigate the effects of the situation.

Team-cooperative families are characterized by a commitment to collective goals. Family activities are undertaken to obtain the goals, with each member of the family having something to contribute. The family members may work together in times of crisis to cope with the situation.

In legal-bureaucratic families, the members respond to each other because it is their duty. Usually one person is in-charge, and compliance is obtained because he or she holds the authority to define how members shall behave. If the family decision-maker is functional, this type of family may organize quickly to deal with a crisis. However, if the authority in the family has resided with the hospice patient, who now is unable to act, the family may have difficulty with decision-making and may expend considerable energy deciding who is now in-charge. Control, who has it and who wants it, is a frequent issue in legal-bureaucratic families.

Families in which bargaining is the prevailing transactional mode use negotiation as the principal method for deciding who shall do what. Each member gives and receives something in return, with the expectation that everyone wins something of value. Frequently, these families possess a flexibility that serves them well in crisis situations. Coercion is the least adaptive family transactional mode since it involves the use of deception, threat, or force. With the exception of coercion, strengths exist in each transactional mode which may be mobilized when a family is experiencing the death of a member.

Subsystems. Subsystems are the component parts of the family. They may be thought of as the individuals who are the family members or as the roles that the members play in the family. The marital and in-law subsystems are formed when a couple marries. The parent-child and grandparent-grandchild subsystems are formed with the birth of the first child, and the sibling subsystem is formed with the birth of a second child. The creation of each new subsystem or the loss of an established one requires a reworking of the relationships within the family. A dysfunctional or absent marital subsystem poses special problems for families. The anticipation of the loss of a spouse is always threatening not only to the marriage partner but also to the children, who if young, may require additional years of parenting, or if mature, may wonder how the death of a parent will influence their relationship with and need to care for the remaining parent.

Boundaries. Boundaries mark the interfaces between the family and its environment and among the family subsystems. External boundaries indicate the outer conceptual or physical limits of the family, thus determining who is "in" and who is "out" of the family. Internal boundaries set the limits which separate the family subsystems. Evidence of internal boundaries may be seen in who speaks to whom, who is cut off from other family members, and how members align themselves along gender and generational lines. Both the external and internal boundaries are semipermeable in that they allow for exchange of matter, energy, and information between the family and its environment and among the various family subsystems.

Philosophy. Philosophy refers to an orientation toward life which guides family decision-making. It is determined by the family values, goals, ideals, religious beliefs, and expectations of life. The family's philosophy may include an explanation for suffering which sustains the members through their experience of loss, or it may be of little assistance to them in anticipation of the death of a loved one. As with all crisis, death offers the opportunity for growth as well as danger (Rapoport, 1965). Anticipation of death gives the patient and family an opportunity for healing the past conflicts and disablements of family living (Ackerman, 1972; Bloomfield, 1983; Friedman, 1985) if they can be helped to use the experience for that purpose. Hospice caregivers have a special opportunity to promote family health at a critical time in the family's history.

Life style. Life style refers to the persistent characteristic behavior of the family members which is encompassed in the family's norms, roles, rules, secrets, myths, traditions, and rituals. A norm is a smallest, single behavioral act that is acceptable for a given interactional situation. Norms provide the standards for behavior as well as the standards for judging behavior (Bertrand, 1972). For example, punctuality may be a norm for a particular family. As long as the norm is met, little notice is given it. Once broken, compliance becomes an issue. Late medications may be viewed as evidence that the staff is incompetent instead of involved in caring for an emergency. Knowing family norms helps the staff predict what behaviors have special meaning for clients and families.

Norms usually occur in clusters, and when taken together they constitute roles. Roles are composed sets of norms dedicated to the same function and having characteristics that permit the prediction of behavior (Bertrand, 1972). An individual performing a certain role exhibits the behaviors expected in the role. Roles may be thought of as dyadic relationships, such as husband-wife, parent-child, nurse-patient, with the hyphen symbolizing the interactional nature of the relationship between the role participants (G.M. Sills, personal communication, 1972). Roles are never enacted in isolation; rather they are negotiated between the role participants (Hart & Herriott, 1985).

Although roles lend predictability, their enactment is always to some extent unique (Hall, 1985b). Thus, what is considered the role of the husband and the wife in a patient's family may be very different from what are expected role behaviors in the family of the professional caregiver. Family members who act in ways which do not meet the role expectations of the hospice staff, may have negotiated their roles very differently from the caregiver's family. It is also possible that the stress of the current situation prevents the patient's family from enacting their roles in their usual manner. The crises of illness and death of a family member always require a change in family roles; hence the importance of the staff's understanding and support while spouses and other family members learn to live without their previous role partners. Supportive care for hospice survivors is crucial even though not reimbursable in many instances. One can become widowed in a very few minutes, but learning the new roles associated with the status requires much longer.

All families have rules, most often unspoken, which are major determinates of a family's life style. Family rules are implicit, unwritten laws which govern family behavior, most often outside the awareness of family members. Ford and Herrick (1974) observed that several rules frequently appear in combination to structure specific family life styles. Examples of family life styles include: the children come first, two against the world, share and share alike, every man for himself, and until death do us part. Undoubtedly, experienced hospice caregivers have developed their own metaphors to identify the family life styles they see in their practice, and only need to make them explicit to assist others in understanding family dynamics.

Family life styles are also influenced by family secrets which are aspects of family history that are known to some members but not to others. The secret often involves a stigmatizing event, such as conception prior to marriage or the existence of a previous marriage that does not become known until hidden family records are examined at the time of a member's death. The family members may grow up totally unaware of the event, or they may have known but have learned from early childhood that certain topics of conversation are taboo. Family secrets are made powerful by their covertness. Rules develop to maintain a conspiracy of silence and deception, thus mystifying family communications.

Family myth is a term used by Ferreira (1963) to indicate a series of well-integrated beliefs shared by family members that go unchallenged in spite of the distortions of reality that they present. Myths are a part of the family's inner image which serve a protective function by hiding a vulnerable aspect of the family. The themes of myths usually deal with issues of family happiness or unhappiness. Examples include "all is well" with the family when relationships are deteriorating, and "we never get angry" when stoney silence shouts otherwise. Family members actively contribute to the myth and strive to preserve it. Even when a member privately may doubt its validity, the individual is under an injunction not to investigate, much less challenge, the myth, for it defends the family image and explains the behavior of the family members.

Family Process

Family processes are series of changes which are arranged in a special order that occur continuously through time, both within the family and between the family and its environment. The purpose of family processes is to maintain the structure and to carry out the functions of the family. Family processes have to do with adaptation, integration, decision-making, information-processing, communication, coalition-formation, conflict management, and commitment (Hall, 1985a). Bredemeier (n.d.) states that adaptation, integration, and decision-making are essential for a social system's survival. The other processes have been incorporated into the conceptual model to describe how a family goes about adaptation, integration, and decision-making.

Adaptation. Adaptation is the two-way process of influencing and being influenced by the environment which occurs at the family-environment boundary. It involves the boundary maintenance functions of obtaining, containing, retaining, and disposing (Sills & Hall, 1985). The family must obtain what it needs from the environment, such as shelter, food, and health care. It also must contain within the environment those influences that are not required or that are detrimental to the family. Examples of such influences include intractable pain, disruptive visitors, and resuscitation measures not desired by the patient.

Family members also work to retain within the family that which it requires to function, such as the right to make decisions concerning its members' health care. Finally, members must dispose of the family's products and what the family no longer needs. Examples include launching functional young adults, dispelling family myths, and disempowering family secrets.

The process of adaptation with the environment is one of the most crucial family survival mechanisms. Assessment of the manner in which the family carries out obtaining, containing, retaining, and disposing tells professional caregivers a great deal about the family's effectiveness and its ability to function in ways appropriate for meeting the needs of its members. The advantage of hospice care is that the environment in which the patient and the family must cope with a terminal illness can be modified to make adaptation easier. For example, the hospice nurse or occupational therapist can work with the family caregiver about how to modify the bathroom to make bathing the ill family member easier and safer.

Hospice team members can also assist the family in modifying a room in the general living area to accommodate a hospital bed, thereby allowing the dying family member to have a view of the garden and be nearer to her family.

> During an initial home visit a woman in her mid-40s with metastatic lung cancer was found laying in a fetal position on her back; she was on the living room sofa. John, her husband, stated that they had moved her downstairs from their bedroom so that she could be more closely monitored. Janet was incontinent of urine, extremely emancipated, and would moan when I tried to relax her legs off of her shoulders. Clearly, John was doing the best that he could, but he was extremely tired from his 24 hours responsibilities which included three children and a full-time job. Fortunately, Janet's parents were retired and had moved into a nearby apartment in order to help John with her care and with the children. I made arrangements to have a hospital bed delivered and to have the sofa moved to another part of the house. I received orders to insert a foley catheter and to put Janet on around the clock pain medication versus prn. The family was instructed on dietary supplements and skin care. Within a couple of days Janet was able to lay flat and she was more responsive to her family.

Most families will need help in modifying the home environment. Yet this time is well spent as illustrated through the words of a bereaved husband following the death of his wife of 47 years: "I hope that the love and flowers and birds and the sense that she was home and not in an institution helped" (Gonda & Ruark, 1984, p. 6). We believe it did.

In some cases, the family may elect not to care for the dying person at home. When this situation occurs and the dying family member is in an in-patient hospice setting the staff can work with the family to adapt the environment to feel more home-like. For example, the family may bring in a comforter, favorite pictures, or the family pet. The hospice staff may also assist the family in disposing of unwanted visitors by limiting the number of people who visit and/or monitoring the time that any one person stays.

Integration. Integration refers to the process by which the family maintains its cohesiveness as a system in order to carry out its functions and achieve its goals. Inevitably, some tension exists between the individual members' needs and desires and the collective goals of the family. Functional families usually find ways to negotiate these differences. However, tension may reach conflict proportions when a family is thrown off balance by terminal illness.

A couple in their early 70s had been dating for 10 years. Prior to becoming terminally ill the older gentleman was very attentive to the needs of his lady friend, he helped her with yardwork, took her dancing frequently, and often shared meals with her. As Mr. Smith's care needs increased he was less able to focus his attention on Miss Johnson and their social activities steadily declined. Upon hospice admission Miss Johnson expressed a great deal of anger at having to care for Mr. Smith and the drastic change in their relationship. On one hand she felt committed to the relationship, on the other hand she needed someone to fill the void his illness had created. The hospice program was unable to meet the multiple needs of this woman despite her repeated attempts to get various team members to take care of her. Although one could view this couple's relationship as having been dysfunctional prior to the illness, clearly Mr. Smith needed to be needed which was reciprocal to Miss Johnson wanting to be taken care of. With the support of the hospice team Miss Johnson was able to care for Mr. Smith during the days before his death and to be with him when he died.

Decision-making. Decision-making is the process of making choices about how to use family resources to carry out adaptation and integration. The process assumes that family members are rational and tend to make optimal choices when faced with alternatives. The process is influenced by the family's goals and philosophy. Decisions also can be profoundly influenced by the stress that family is experiencing. During crises, decisions may not appear rational. Heretofore unacknowledged family values may come into play, prioritizing options according to emotional needs rather than logic. The executive function (decision-making) of the family may be compromised, thus requiring support and understanding from care providers. The case of a family from Africa whose 18 year old daughter died of cancer serves to illustrate this point.

> The family had lived in the United States for the majority of the daughter's life and she and her siblings were enculturated, however the mother continued to dress according to the cultural norms of her native country and both parents frequently conversed in their native language. Following the diagnosis of cancer, Mary was transferred from the teaching hospital to a private in-patient hospice unit to spend the last weeks of her life. At the time of her death I was present with the majority of family and a hospice social worker. Mary's brother had returned to college, his father promised that Mary would be alright and that he could see her on the weekend. The brother was contacted at school late in the evening on the night of Mary's death; his friends drove him 150 miles to the hospice unit.
>
> Although some of the staff had talked about how this death and the family's response could differ, the real impact of the native culture had not been fully acknowledged. When Mary died her parents expressed their desire to take her body with them, a request that was viewed as highly atypical. Between the time of Mary's death at midnight and 6:00 a.m. we stayed with the family in order to problem solve how to proceed. In the end, a funeral home was selected and they came to remove Mary's body from the facility. The situation had a profound

impact on the staff as we processed our role in meeting the needs of the family. The parents experienced not only the death of their daughter that evening, but they also experienced a lack of understanding of cultural diversity. As the nurse in attendance at the death I viewed the parents as unable to make appropriate decisions, when in fact Mary's parents were responding to the stress in a way that was familiar and comfortable to them.

Information-processing. Information-processing is obtaining and using information to create and maintain the family's structure and to carry out the other family processes. It is closely related to decision-making since it supplies the data upon which the family acts. Frequently a family's need for information goes undetected; without reliable data, families cannot be expected to make effective decisions. Also, there are times when families can not process what is being told them, because their anxiety prevents them from hearing and using the information. Later, they may deny that they were given certain information. Therefore, it is important to assess not only what a family needs and has a right to know, but also what they are capable of dealing with at the moment.

Communication. Communication is the process of giving and receiving meaning, including verbal and nonverbal behavior, symbols, clues and cues. It is closely related to information-processing and necessary for decision-making. Therapeutic communication is a major intervention strategy of caring for people. The sense of having been heard, the feeling that someone understands, and the knowledge that someone cares is profoundly healing.

Presumedly, meaningful relationships are based on a sense of love and trust. However, a great deal of what goes on between people in family relationships does not always convey positive feelings. Consequently, people develop alternatives to use as survival methods when that happens. Satir (1975) has identified five modes which families use to communicate or avoid communicating their feelings during times of stress. These include placating, blaming, super-reasonableness, irrelevance, and congruence.

Placating communications are those that soothe feelings by concession or giving in to the other person, while disregarding one's own feelings, wishes, or opinions. Agreement is stated when it does not exist, and the feeling of being compromised persists far beyond the interaction. Placating may be a long standing pattern in the family, with one or several persons consistently giving in to another. Or placating may be a way that both family members and staff deal with a patient whom they believe is too ill to be held to the usual standards of behavior.

Blaming is another mechanism that people have of dealing with situations. People blame when they feel powerless and need to shift the burden of their feelings of inadequacy. Thus, the staff may be blamed because the course of the patient's illness cannot be reversed. Family members who hold unrealistic self-expectations may blame themselves for not being able to care for the patient at home. Others may blame God for their own or their loved one's worsening condition. Children frequently misinterpret situations that they are too young to understand. Believing, or being told, that they are responsible for a parent's illness is an awesome burden. The guilt which develops may color a person's entire life.

Some persons tend to intellectualize and become super-reasonable when communicating under stress. While their words are logical, they bear no relationship to what the persons are actually feeling. These people have learned that it is dangerous to reveal their feelings. Their lack of expression gives the impression that they are not fully present in the situation or that they really do not care what happens. Such people may resort to super-reasonableness when they are afraid to show their emotions for they have never learned how to be tender and comforting with others. Often they fear that the loss of composure will render them ineffective and unable to act.

Some people's conversation becomes totally irrelevant under stress. A patient may say that she is dying, only to be asked by her visitors where she went on her last vacation. The listeners' discomfort is so intense that they dare not acknowledge what the patient is saying. Unable to deal with the intensity of their own feelings, they change the subject to distract the patient from discussing what may be most meaningful to her. Other people may chatter incessantly so that no one has a chance to bring up emotionally loaded topics, thus blocking meaningful communications.

The need for these four communication modes is understandable and everyone uses them from time to time. However, a fifth method, congruence, is more functional (Satir, 1975). Congruence in communication occurs when the person's thoughts, feelings, words and nonverbal behaviors match and thus the message he or she sends is clearly understood. If a patient is in pain but his words deny it while his position indicates it, the listener is left with a mixed message that requires clarification. Valuable time is lost in providing for his comfort and perhaps he will never receive what he needs. The achievement of congruence in communication is difficult for some people because they have learned not to say what they are really thinking or feeling. They may have grown up in a family in which one of the unspoken rules was "don't say what you feel." They have yet to learn that relationships can survive the expression of strong emotions and be strengthened by congruence in communications.

Coalition-formation. Coalition-formation is the process by which people align themselves for the purpose of achieving their goals. Coalitions form within families, within groups of health care-providers, and between providers and family members. Some coalitions are to be fostered, such as a therapeutic relationship between patients and caregivers and supportive relationships among family members. Other coalitions need to be evaluated to determine their therapeutic effect. Covert coalitions, those which people try to keep hidden, always raise the question of why does the relationship need to be secret.

Conflict management. Conflict management is concerned with the constructive use of the conflict that inevitably arises in families and sometimes develops between families and professional caregivers. Conflict frequently is viewed from a negative perspective as a condition always to be avoided. A more balanced view recognizes that conflict can have constructive or destructive effects, depending upon how the family deals with it. Conflict is the natural result of differences in philosophy and lifestyle preferences among the family members and between the family and other systems with which they interact. Mismatches in transactional modes sometimes give rise to conflict between the family and health care workers. The family may be very Gemeinschaft in its interactions, while health care providers are accustomed to working in legal-bureaucratic environments. These differences may require negotiation. The aim of conflict management is to find a creative solution to problems arising from divergent views.

Commitment. Commitment is the process by which family members are dedicated to and invested in each other. It involves loyalty and ongoing mutual support which grows out of loving concern for the welfare of others. Commitment can also be observed in hospice workers' relationships with patients and families and as well as with each other. Demonstrating caring concern for the terminally ill can be physically and emotionally taxing for families and professional caregivers alike. Families need respite care, and the staff requires a source of ongoing support to remain capable of dealing with the stressful situations which characterize their practice.

In summary, the family as a system can be conceptualized as having both structural and process components which may be a locus of the family's strengths and/or limitations. These components serve as one of the two major constructs basic to family assessment and intervention. The second major construct is the family life cycle, which draws from family developmental theory.

Family Life Cycle

Carter and McGoldrick (1988) conceptualize the family life cycle as encompassing the entire three- or four-generation system as it moves through six stages of development. They hold the view that stress is often the greatest during transition from one developmental stage to another, and that family dysfunction is most likely to appear when there is an interruption or dislocation in the natural timing of the family life cycle. The developmental stages in which a family experiences a death is significant in determining the influence the death will have on family members.

Stage I: Between Families –
Single Young Adult

Each of the six family development stages include changes in the family structure that involve shifts in the family's boundaries. The first of the six stages of the family life cycle, the launching period, requires the young adult to leave adolescence and to function as an adult at college or in the world of work. Career choices and intimacy issues are of central importance. Relationships must be reworked with the family of origin, the task of the parent being to let go and the task of the young adult to move from dependency to independence. For young adults, this is a period of trying on new behaviors as they develop their own philosophy and life style.

> Mary and her family were at this stage in their development. Mary and her twin sister, Ann, had both graduated from high school and were to start college in the fall. Mary's plans changed when her advanced cancer was diagnosed during exploratory surgery in the summer. She delayed starting college in the fall but planned to join her sister for the winter term. Ann did start college in the fall; she believed that Mary would get well. Mary died that fall. Ann returned to college following the funeral, however her desire to share her college days with her twin was never fulfilled.

Stage II: Joining of Families
Through Marriage

When families are joined through marriage in the second stage of the family life cycle, the new couple must work out mutual positions on many issues which they previously had decided individually or in a manner dictated by their families of origin. Becoming established as a couple requires major boundary realignments. The couple exists as a new family, separate yet related to their extended families. The in-law subsystem is established, with the parents continuing the task of letting go. Issues of separateness and togetherness are paramount between the marriage partners and between the couple and their families of origin.

Stage III: Families with Young Children

Becoming parents marks the beginning of the third family developmental stage. The birth of a child brings about profound change in the nuclear and extended family (Bradt, 1988) and requires a reworking of household routines, leisure activities, work commitments, and relationships with the new grandparents and other members of the extended family. The birth of a second child creates the sibling subsystem, adding further complexity to the family structure.

> Janet and John were a family with young children when they were referred to hospice. After they married they adopted their first child, which was followed by the birth of two children. Janet stopped working and became very involved in the work of the home and raising the children. Prior to her illness she was president of the PTA and enjoyed playing golf. Janet lived just under two years from the time of initial diagnosis and her children ranged in age from 8 to 13 years at the time of her death. Janet's death meant that John was without a wife and the mother of his children, something he nor his children ever acknowledged as a possibility prior to Janet's illness.

Stage IV: Families with Adolescents

Families with adolescents is the fourth stage of family development. As Preto (1988) notes, the adolescent's maturing sense of identity and autonomy demands structural shifts in the family and the renegotiation of roles involving at least three generations of relatives. Further complexity is added to the family system by the developmental tasks of the middlescent parents who are faced with accepting their own maturing years and the prospect of coming to terms with their own parents. Blenker (1965) uses the term filial maturity to describe that point in the middle years when individuals first see their parents as real people, with all the strengths and limitations that being human implies. Thus, relationships are being reworked at multiple levels during this stage of family development.

Stage V: Families Launching Children

Launching children is the major focus of the fifth stage of family development. The child's exit from the nuclear family creates a new family in the first stage of development, that of the single adult who is between his family of origin and the establishment of a family of procreation (Stage I). Again, the transitions have to do with shifts in family boundaries, both internal and external, and with the renegotiation of family roles.

McCullough and Rutenberg (1988) have identified four transitions and related developmental tasks during this stage of family development. These include the changing function of marriage from procreation to companionship, development of adult-to-adult relationships between parents and their grown children, the expansion of family relationships to include in-laws and grandchildren, and the opportunity to resolve unfinished business with aging parents. This is a period of multiple opportunities for family peacemaking as the middle-aged person reworks relationships with his or her spouse or significant other, adult children, and aging parents (Hall & Peterson, 1989). The movies, *The Gathering* (Barera, Sherman & Kleisei, 1977) and *On Golden Pond* (Gilbert & Rydell, 1981), illustrate how selected families approached family peacemaking.

Most couples lose one or more parents at this time. This loss is frequently preceded by a period in which the middlescent adult manages or gives direct care to a parent. It is also a time when families are likely to need hospice care. With the high incidence of chronic disease during the middle years, the members of the middle generation may find that they are dealing with their own health problems in addition to those of a terminally ill parent.

Stage VI: Families in Later Life

The family in the latter years describes the final stage of the family life cycle (Walsh, 1988). Family life during the latter years is marked by a series of losses. Spouses, friends, siblings and extended family members die. The remaining spouse may remarry or have years of living alone with reliance on children and grandchildren for support. While not inevitable, failing health and dependency may strain the physical, emotional, and financial resources of adult children.

Developmental Influences

Hospice caregivers may be called upon to assist families at all stages of the family life cycle. The stage in which the death occurs determines the family and individual developmental tasks which are most likely to be interrupted. The death of a parent may stall the launching of the young adult, making it difficult for him or her to establish a separate existence. The death of a spouse in young families has a profound effect not only on the marriage partner but also on the quality of the parenting available for young children. Death of a child is especially hard for families to accept, for parents do not expect to bury their young as was common in past generations. Although the unexpected, off-schedule death is often the most stressful, even the expected death of a grandparent can be difficult for the family. Regardless of the stage of the family life cycle or whether the death was expected or unexpected, a death reverberates through the entire system.

The Components of Practice

Each helping discipline has identifiable components of practice which comprise the therapeutic process its practitioners employ when working with families. These components comprise the third dimension of the conceptual framework. The emphasis in the following discussion is how the components of practice serve as the vehicle for the therapeutic application of knowledge of the family as a system and the family life cycle.

Assessment

Assessment consists of the collection and analysis of data about families essential to planning and implementing their care. This can be done in a number of ways, including listening to family communications, direct observation of family interactions, and formalized family history taking. The genogram is useful to record family data obtained by these means. A genogram is a diagrammatic representation of family structure and process which records family data in a compact manner. Visualization of family information in this manner assists in the identification of family patterns, the understanding of which is basic to planning supportive family care. Figure 2 is a beginning genogram for Janet's family described in the previous clinical example. It is interesting to note the lack of information about John's family of origin; John did not talk about his family with the hospice staff and the information was not systematically assessed.

The construction of a genogram can be commenced by the staff from the moment of the first contact with the family, and further elaborations are accomplished as family data becomes available. Families and patients, if able, frequently find comfort in actively assisting in the construction of their family's genogram. The genogram is an effective instrument for securing sensitive family data

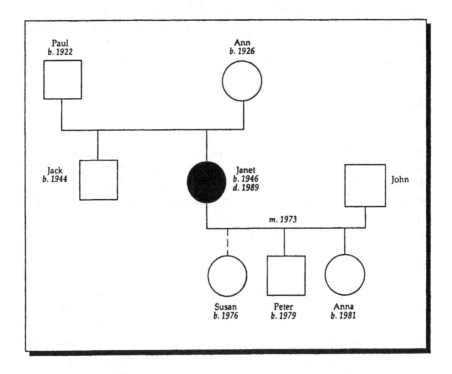

Figure 2. Family genogram.

without arousing undue anxiety (McGoldrick & Gerson, 1985). Families have the opportunity to identify their strengths and how support can be engendered for the patient. If family problems exist, furnishing historical data for a genogram permits the family members to "tell their story" to a non-judgmental listener. Frequently, such discussions give family members new insights about their family. Assessment is never just assessment. It always contains some element of intervention, for the process of giving the family history changes the person's understanding of that history. Observing family relationships visually represented on a genogram can be as informative to the patient and the family as it is to the care provider.

The drawing of genograms can be accomplished manually and recorded on the patient's chart where all members of the hospice care team have access to them. If the patient and family actively participate in the construction of the genogram, the original drawing should be large enough for them to see. Blackboards or large sheets of butcher paper can serve this purpose. Genograms can also be computer-generated with the aid of several programs developed by Gerson (1984, 1989). Family members may wish to have a copy of their genogram. Often they add or correct information while the family is receiving hospice services (not at all in a facility).

Planning

The development of mutually agreed upon family and patient care goals is a natural extension of joint construction of the family genogram. The family and the patient who are actively involved in the development of the plan of care are likely to feel more in control of their lives and more able to enter into a partnership with the staff to make the most creative possible use of the hospice experience. Joint planning facilitates implementation of the therapeutic regime recommended by the staff, while meeting the individualized needs of the family.

Intervention

The major focus of intervention with families in hospice care is assisting families to deal with the multiple losses they experience. Duhl (1964) notes five kinds of changes or threats of change which involve loss and which may precipitate a crisis for individuals and families. There are changes in the significant social network, physical environment, body image, psychological self, and beliefs, values, and expectations. The hospice family is faced with all of these changes.

The most threatening change is the death of one of a family's members. Herriott (1982) has identified five factors which determine how persons respond to the termination of a relationship. These include the significance of the relationship, the perceived reliance, previous experiences with separation, investment in alternative relationships, and the timing of the experience.

The significance of the relationship refers to the meaning the deceased person had for the other family members. Under usual conditions one would expect a wife to have a stronger reaction to the death of her husband than one would to the death of a second cousin. For further discussion of the meaning of relationships see Kirschling (1989). Self-reliance has to do with the extent to which the survivors' possess the ability to function without the missing family member and availability of someone to perform the role functions of the deceased member. The nature of the survivors' past experience with separation can help or hinder the current adaptation. Present losses can reactivate unresolved grief making the current situation more difficult, but also presenting family members with an opportunity to resolve past as well as current broken attachments. The extent to which there are alternative relationships available for support also influences a family's response to loss. Timing, whether the death was expected or unexpected, whether it occurred with the usual time table or off schedule, whether the death was viewed as preventable, and in what family developmental stage the death occurs are additional factors that affect how persons respond to the termination of a relationship.

While other losses may be considered of lesser importance, when they are combined with changes in the family's significant social network, they profoundly influence the family. Strangers become important to the family because as caregivers they may be an extension or substitute for family care. Changes in the appearance of the patient and the paraphernalia of physical care may distress the family to an even greater extent than they do the patient. The individual in the bed may no longer look like the person that family members have known for a lifetime. Not only may the patient not appear the same, he or she may not act the same.

> When Janet was admitted to the inpatient hospice unit her mother brought a picture of her for the staff to see. In the staff's eyes Janet was a dying woman who had lost all of her hair and weighed less then 80 pounds. In her family's eyes Janet was a healthy mother, wife and daughter who had shoulder length hair and a beautiful smile. The two images of the same woman were drastically different.

Family members may require assistance in understanding the psychological changes the patient and they themselves are experiencing. Subtle losses must be grieved. The anticipation of death calls for revision in dreams unlived and goals unreached. These are often the unspoken loses which a family faces.

The three balancing factors in crisis situations identified by Aguilera and Messick (1985) as crucial to successful resolution are the perception of the event, coping mechanisms, and situational support. Families are able to deal with their losses to the extent that they hold realistic perceptions of their situations, possess appropriate coping mechanisms, and are afforded adequate situational support. The hospice team can assist families through therapeutic listening to families' perceptions of their experience, giving factual information as appropriate, teaching new coping skills, and mobilizing social support. Thus, the three factors serve both as an assessment and as an intervention guide.

Evaluation

Evaluation of family care can be measured in terms of the family's satisfaction and how well the goals of the family care plan were met. Programs for family care in hospice setting need to be formalized, with specific program objectives, against which the success of the program can be measured.

CONCLUSION

The conceptual framework for caring for families of hospice patients accents the complexity of family-based care. The purpose of this article was to sensitize the reader to the family as client. We would encourage hospice team members to use the framework as a vehicle for identifying relevant family information and as a backdrop for discussing family-based intervention. Given the heterogeneity of the hospice population it is unrealistic to expect that information will be collected from every family and on every concept. However, hospice team members need to be cognizant of the multiple concepts that are involved when the family is viewed as client. The conceptual framework could also be used in hospice training programs, with additional case study material being incorporated, followed by small group discussion. Finally, we would recommend that the conceptual framework be used as vehicle for reflection. The opportunity to revisit and reflect on the three cases described in this article was invaluable. Time for reflection allows the clinician to identify the positive, as well as the negative, aspects of his or her work with a particular family and to identify potential areas for future professional growth.

REFERENCES

Ackerman, N.W. (1972). The growing edge of family therapy. In C.J. Sager & H.S. Kaplan (Eds.), *Progress in group and family therapy* (pp. 440-441). New York: Brunner/Mazel.

Aguilera, D.C., & Messick, J.M. (1985). *Crisis intervention: Theory and methodology*. St. Louis: Mosby.

Barera, J. (Executive Producer), Sherman, H.R. (Producer), & Kleisei, R. (Director). (1977). *The Gathering* [Film]. Los Angeles, CA: Hanna-Barbera Productions.

Bertrand, A. (1972). *Social organization: A general systems and role theory perspective*. Arlington Heights, IL: AHM Publishing.

Blenker, M. (1965). Social work and family relationships in later life with some thoughts on filial maturity. In E. Shanes & G.F. Streib (Eds.), *Social structure and the family*. Englewood Cliffs: Prentice-Hall.

Bloomfield, H.H. (1983). *Making peace with your parents*. New York: Random House.

Bradt, J.O. (1988). Becoming parents: Families with young children. In B. Carter

& M. McGoldrick (Eds.), *The changing family life cycle: A framework for family therapy* (pp. 235-254). New York: Gardner Press.

Bredemeier, H.C. (n.d.). *Social systems: Integration and adaptation.* Unpublished manuscript, Rutgers University, New Brunswick, NJ.

Burgess, E.W., & Locke, H.J. (1953). *The family: From institution to companionship.* New York: American Book.

Carter, B., & McGoldrick, M. (1988). Overview: The changing family life cycle. In B. Carter & M. McGoldrick (Eds.), *The changing family life cycle: A framework for family therapy* (pp. 3-28). New York: Gardner Press.

Duhl, F.J. (1964). *Grief.* Paper presented at the Ohio League of Nursing Convention, Columbus, OH.

Ferreira, A.J. (1963). Family myth and homeostasis. *Archives of General Psychiatry, 9,* 457-463.

Ford, F.R., & Herrick, J. (1974). Family rules: Family life style. *American Journal of Orthopsychiatry, 44*(1), 61-69.

Friedman, E.H. (1985). *Generation to generation: Family process in church and synagogue.* New York: Guilford Press.

Gerson, R. (1984). *The family-data base manager.* Wakefield, RI: Applied Innovations.

Gerson, R. (1989). *MacGenogram: A graphic utility for producing genograms.* Atlanta: Humanware.

Gilbert, B. (Producer), & Rydell, M. (Director). (1981). *On Golden Pond.* [Film]. New York, NY: ITC Films Incorporated.

Gonda, T.A., & Ruark, J. E. (1984). *Dying dignified the health professional's guide to care.* Menlo Park, CA: Addison-Wesley.

Hall, J.E. (1985a). Conceptual basis for nursing practice with complex organizations. In J.E. Hall & B.R. Weaver (Eds.), *Distributive nursing practice: A systems approach to community health* (pp. 212-243). Philadelphia: Lippincott.

Hall, J.E. (1985b). Social organization. In J.E. Hall & B.R. Weaver (Eds.), *Distributive nursing practice: A systems approach to community health* (pp. 30-43). Philadelphia: Lippincott.

Hall, J.E., & Peterson, W. (1989). *Middlescent transition: Making peace with aging parents.* Unpublished manuscript, Oregon Health Sciences University, Portland, OR.

Hart, S.K., & Herriott, P.R. (1985). Components of nursing practice: A systems approach. In J.E. Hall & B.R. Weaver (Eds.), *Distributive nursing practice: A systems approach to community health* (pp. 102-123). Philadelphia: Lippincott.

Herriott, P. (1982). *Termination of the nurse-patient relationship.* Unpublished manuscript.

Kirschling, J.M. (1989). Analysis of Bugen's Model of Grief. *The Hospice Journal, 5*(1), 55-75.

McCullough, P.G., & Rutenberg, S.K. (1988). Launching children and moving on. In B. Carter & M. McGoldrick (Eds.), *The changing family life cycle: A framework for family therapy* (pp. 185-309). New York: Gardner Press.

McCormack, P. (1974, August 4). New family definitions from future leaders. *Sarasota Herald-Tribune.* Sarasota, FL.

McGoldrick, M., & Gerson, R. (1985). *Genograms in family assessment.* New York: Norton.

Preto, N.G. (1988). Transformation of the family system in adolescence. In B. Carter & M. McGoldrick (Eds.), *The changing family life cycle: A framework for family therapy* (pp. 255-283). New York: Gardner Press.

Rapoport, L. (1965). The state of crisis: Some theoretical considerations. In H.J. Parad (Ed.), *Crisis intervention: Selected readings* (pp. 22-31). New York: Family Service Association of America.

Satir, V. (1975). You as a change agent. In V. Satir, J. Stachowiak, & H.A. Tascgman (Eds.), *Helping families to change* (pp. 37-62). New York: Aronson.

Sills, G.M., & Hall, J.E. (1985). A general systems perspective for nursing practice. In J.E. Hall & B.R. Weaver (Eds.), *Distributive nursing practice: A systems approach to community health* (pp. 21-29). Philadelphia: Lippincott.

Terkelson, K.B. (1980). Toward a theory of the family life cycle. In E.A. Carter, & M. McGoldrick (Eds.), *The family life cycle: A framework for family therapy* (pp. 21-52). New York: Gardner Press.

Walsh, F. (1988). The family in later years. In Carter B. & M. McGoldrick (Eds.), *The family life cycle: A framework for family therapy* (pp. 311-332). New York: Gardner Press.

Sources of Stress
for Hospice Caregiving Families

Margaret M. Hull

SUMMARY. The purpose of this qualitative study was to generate a detailed description of the concerns and stresses families encountered as they cared for their dying relative in an oncology hospice home care program. Semi-structured interviews and participant observation were used to follow 14 family members from 10 different families throughout their caregiving experiences. The constant comparative method of data analysis was used to discover emergent themes. Families identified three general sources of stress: patient symptoms, interactions with others, and concerns for self. Findings were examined from within the larger body of caregiving literature. Changes in their relatives' mental status seemed most stressful over time, and is an area that may benefit from increased support from health professionals.

Hospice home care of a dying relative is a rapidly growing alternative to traditional hospital based terminal care for patients with cancer. The number of hospices in the United States increased from one in 1971 to currently over 1700 fully operational programs (National Hospice Organization [NHO], 1988). With the predominant focus of home care, families play a vital role in providing the day to

Margaret M. Hull, PhD, RN, is Assistant Professor at The Ohio State University College of Nursing, Department of Life Span Process, 1585 Neil Ave., Columbus, OH 43210-1289. Dr. Hull has worked with hospice patients and their family caregivers in both home care and in-patient settings. Her research focus is on family caregivers undertaking hospice supported home care.

This research was supported by the Department of Health and Human Services, National Center for Nursing Research, National Research Service Award Predoctoral Fellowship F31 NR05831-03 and The American Cancer Society, New York State Division Pre-doctoral Fellowship.

day care for their dying relatives. Within the past decade, family caregiving has been the focus of major research attention. Areas of investigation include (a) characteristics of caregivers and care recipients; (b) tasks of caregiving; (c) impact of caregiving on the caregiver, especially the frail elderly; and (d) impact of caregiving for a relative with senile dementia or Alzheimer's disease. Except for studies that focused on caring for the cognitively impaired, caregiving has not been examined within specific medical diagnoses. It seems that some needs, concerns, difficulties and stresses may be closely related to the course and treatment of a given illness and that caring for a dying relative with a cancer versus a non-cancer illness might be a different experience. In addition, hospice care is offered for the last 6 months of life. Examining caregiving that involved a relatively short term commitment rather than the longer involvements typically noted in the caregiving literature may add information to this body of knowledge. However, far less is known about the caregiving experiences of hospice home care families whose relative is dying of cancer. Therefore, examination of caregiving within hospice as a home care alternative seems warranted.

Previous nursing research with families caring for a terminally ill relative at home has focused on two variables, family needs and the supportiveness of nursing behaviors. Of most importance to families was knowledge about their relatives' conditions, prognosis, and signs of imminent death (Garland, Bass, & Otto, 1984; Googe & Varricchio, 1981; Skorupka & Bohnet, 1982). Assurance about their relatives' comfort and adequacy of pain control also were of primary concern (McGinnis, 1986; Skorupka & Bohnet). Learning needs regarding these measures as well as ambulation techniques were identified by home care families (Grobe, Ilstrup, & Ahmann 1981; Hinds, 1985).

Within these studies families were asked to respond to multiple item inventories developed by the researchers. Content validity was well established through the use of extensive literature reviews and consultations with experts in the areas of oncology, death and dying, loss, and hospice care. However, families' experiences were rarely used to generate descriptive items included in the research tools. Rather, families were asked to respond to statements others felt to be appropriate for them during their relatives' terminal illnesses. Though these studies were helpful in initial identification of caregivers' areas of concern, the cross-sectional approach limited understanding of this clinical problem to one point in time during the terminal period. Since the duration of the terminal experience encompasses more than a single instance, it is expected that the perspectives of family caregivers will change over time and be affected by personal, environmental, and social influences related to their own situation and also their relatives' changing conditions. Use of a cross-sectional design has not addressed the dynamic nature of this experience over time, within the social context in which it occurs, and limits the ability to understand the full nature of what families deal with. Allowing family members to generate this information from their own life situations as they go about caring for their dying relatives at home will enhance our understanding of what this experience is like for them. Subsequently, health care professionals can begin to develop interventions for further investigation based on families' accounts of the concerns and stresses they confront as caregivers for their dying relatives. Therefore, the purpose of this study was to generate a detailed description of the concerns and stresses families encountered as they cared for their dying relatives within an oncology hospice home care program.

METHOD

A longitudinal qualitative methodology combining semi-structured interviews and participant observation was used to examine the subjective reality of this experience from the participants' points of view. Multiple home visits were conducted with each caregiving family in order to observe caring within the context in which it occurred. Frequency of visits was determined primarily by changes in patients' conditions. If there was stability in the caregiving experience, visits were made every 3 to 4 weeks. If changes in patients' conditions occurred, or changes in caregivers' circumstances or experiences were indicated, more frequent visits were made. Phone contact with the hospice nurses as well as with families was used to gather information that could be used to assess changes that warranted a visit.

Setting and Sample

This study was conducted in an oncology hospice program in a large northeastern city. Home care was the major focus of this program, though five inpatient beds were available at a free-standing unit (FSU). This facility was used primarily to offer short term respite for caregivers or for acute symptom control. Hospice census was maintained at 30-35 patients. To be eligible for the study, family members had to have a relative enrolled in the hospice program, be 18 years of age or older, and able to understand and speak English. Participants could be the primary caregiver in the home, any other adult living in the home with or without care responsibilities for their dying relative, or any adult living outside the home who had consistent patient care responsibilities. The variety of family members was an attempt to examine the extent to which the caregiving experience impacted on all family members, rather than a single primary caregiver.

Staff nurses introduced the study to eligible families on a routine home care visit and left a copy of the consent. This consent contained detailed information on the purpose of the study, what participation involved, and the risks and benefits of participation. The investigator made phone contact with families within two days to discuss any questions and elicit participation.

Fourteen individual family members from 10 different families were enrolled. Seven families contributed a single family member, the primary caregiver (PCG). Two families contributed two family members, the primary caregiver and her spouse. One family contributed three family members, a father and son who alternated the role of PCG, and a daughter who lived out of state and served as PCG during periodic visits over the course of her mother's illness. Relationship of caregivers and patients varied. Six children were caring for a parent, 4 wives and 1 husband were caring for their spouse, 2 sons-in-law were helping to care for their wife's parent, and 1 niece was caring for her aunt. Ages of caregivers ranged from 26 to 78. Ages of patients ranged from 41 to 90. Table 1 displays ages and relationships of caregivers and their dying relatives.

TABLE 1. Age and Relationship of Caregivers and Patients

CAREGIVER			PATIENT	
		AGE and RELATIONSHIP		
40 year old wife		caring for	41 year old husband	
49	wife		54	husband
75	wife		85	husband
78	wife		85	husband
64	daughter		83	mother
40	niece		69	aunt
26	son		65	father
40	daughter &		75	mother/
41	son-in-law		75	mother-in-law
49	daughter &		90	father/
50	son-in-law		90	father-in-law
75	husband,		70	wife/
35	son &		70	mother/
37	daughter		70	mother

Procedures for Data Collection

At the first interview written informed consent was obtained from each participant. Permission to tape record the interviews was given by all subjects. All data were kept confidential. Interviews were conducted in the home. Privacy was easily maintained because patients were out of the home for short periods, napping, or in their rooms. Caregivers were assured that interruptions to maintain patient care responsibilities were expected and would not be a problem for the investigator. This was often a time when participant observation was possible.

When more than one family member participated in the study, the first interview was conducted with both subjects present. Families seemed more comfortable together for this initial visit. Subsequent interviews were conducted individually to encourage more open communication.

Specific questions were addressed on the first interview. These included: What concerns do you have that are specifically related to caring for your dying relative? In what areas of your life do you feel you need more help/understanding/information? What are the most difficult parts about caring for your relative at home? What symptoms are most difficult for you to deal with? Once structured content on the interview guide had been addressed, following interviews were more open-ended. Initial interviews were 2-3 hours after which a flexible schedule of informal visits and interviews was established with each family. Subsequent interviews averaged 60-90 minutes. Field observations were taped immediately after each visit to assure accuracy and thoroughness of the investigator's impressions. Typed transcriptions of interviews and field observations were made and clarified by listening to the tapes while reading the transcriptions.

A final interview was conducted 3 weeks after the patient died and served several purposes: it allowed the researcher to extend her sympathies for the family's loss in person, thank them for sharing their experience, and establish closure. Final interviews were conducted with 13 family members in 9 of the 10 study families: 12 family members whose relative died, and 1 son who withdrew his father from hospice to pursue a day care program of occupational and physical therapy. One patient was alive at the end of data collection and continued in the hospice program under his wife's care.

In summary, 55 visits were made over 16 months of data collection. Total time families were enrolled in hospice ranged from 2.5 to 31 months. Prior to enrollment in the study, families had been involved in the hospice program anywhere from 1 to 26 months. Participation in the study lasted from 1 to 12 months. Visits per family ranged from 2 to 10.

Data Analysis

The constant comparative method of content analysis of transcribed interviews and field notes involved coding for themes emerging over the course of data collection (Glaser, 1978; Glaser &

Strauss, 1967). Phrases, sentences, or anecdotes that represented individual thoughts, feelings, or concepts were separated into relevant themes. Coded data were clustered into categories that described and explained phenomena. Categories were compared with each other to discover conceptual and theoretical linkages between them. Related categories were merged and reduced and new categories were added. Saturation of data occurred when new categories ceased to emerge and no different responses or observations were obtained. Throughout this process codes, i.e., conceptual labels, were assigned to data at all levels of abstraction. Recurrent themes became evident as single words or short phrases were coded and analyzed for similar content. Often, subjects' words or ideas were used to identify this latter group of categories.

Analytic notes had been made throughout data collection and reflected thoughts and questions suggested by the coding process, thus allowing openness to additional ideas. These notes served several functions. First, they facilitated recording and organizing results of the analysis. Second, analytic notes indicated what ground the investigator had covered and what directions were necessary to explore as the research progressed. Finally, analytic notes were the basis for writing the findings (Corbin, 1986).

Validation and Verification of Data

Since the purposes, goals and world views of qualitative research differ from those of the more traditional quantitative research, several authors have suggested more appropriate standards by which to evaluate the scientific merit or rigor of qualitative studies. Sandelowski (1986) suggested several strategies for achieving rigor in qualitative research based on the work of Guba and Lincoln (1981). Four factors compose this framework: credibility, applicability, consistency, and confirmability.

Credibility, or truth value is established when those individuals who were the focus of the investigation immediately recognize themselves and their experience in the descriptions and interpretations of the phenomenon. In addition, credibility occurs when readers other than the researcher or the subjects recognize the described experience. In this study, credibility was addressed in two ways.

First, subjects were asked to comment on the "truth" of the findings as described and to confirm interpretations the researcher made from their experiences. Second, several individuals not involved in this study were asked to review the findings and comment on their ability to recognize the described experience.

Applicability or fittingness, refers to the ability to "fit" findings into the data from which they originated. Findings should reflect typical and atypical aspects of the experience. Recurrent patterns and themes addressed typical aspects. Atypical phenomena were noted and often were helpful in clarifying categories and directing more abstract theoretical linkages of these categories. The analysis process also included independent analysis of segments of the data by colleagues to support and validate the applicability of the investigator's findings. Discussions of colleagues' impressions led to additional questions to be asked of families as well as of current data. Analytic notes recorded these questions.

Consistency, or auditability of qualitative research is achieved when the "decision trail" used by the researcher can be followed by others to arrive at similar conclusions given the data, researcher's framework, and situation. Meeting this criterion involves detailed description of each phase of the research project. Again, independent analysis of portions of the data by colleagues was conducted. Auditability can best be evaluated from written reports of the study.

Confirmability refers to findings that emerge from a research process that values the subjective involvement of researcher and subject while emphasizing the meanings subjects attribute to and derive from their life situations. Confirmability is assured when the three previous criteria are met.

FINDINGS

Findings from this study need to be viewed from within the context of the sample studied and should not be considered as universal for hospice family caregivers. Rather, these findings should be utilized as a means of learning more about their experiences. Information obtained from this research can assist in the generation of substantive theory and research regarding this understudied and rapidly growing group of caregivers.

One additional comment regarding these findings is related to the notion of process and change over time. The initial purpose to examine change over time is less evident in these findings specific to the stresses families experienced. This data is part of a larger study that focused on family caregiving from initial recognition of the terminal nature of their relatives' conditions, through investigation of terminal care alternatives, to immersion in the caregiving role, to 3 weeks after their relatives' deaths. The specific stresses described were part of immersion into the caregiving role. Though families did experience stress in earlier phases of caregiving, they spent far more time and energy describing the following stresses.

Family members identified three general areas of stress that were present throughout their caregiving experience: patient symptoms; interactions with others, i.e., nuclear and extended family members, friends, and personal care aides; and concerns for self.

Patient Symptoms

For many families the most distressing symptoms were those related to changes in their relatives' mental status: inability to communicate, confusion, and seizure activity. In addition, physical deterioration of their relatives' conditions brought about dependence on caregivers for very basic and personal activities of daily living (ADLs).

As patients began to demonstrate decreasing mental acuity, normal interaction patterns were no longer possible. The means by which patients expressed their unique personalities were absent. Family members found themselves interacting on a very simple and rudimentary level with individuals who often were unable to respond in their usual manner, or at all.

> You know, it's the matters that I can't share with him. The thing is, if it were something I could share with him, it's not that I could enjoy it, but I think it would be more tolerable. Up to now he's been relatively in no pain, but not lucid. Then you've got the person who's in terrible pain and lucid. Now I don't know which one's better. I imagine for him it's better

this way, but for all of us—I mean we just can't share it. He just doesn't understand that I want to talk to him. He's just not processing. (40 year old wife)

She insists that there are things that are here (that shouldn't be). She came up with an extra pair of scissors yesterday. They weren't mine and they were in her sewing drawer. She would just say that they weren't hers. It doesn't make sense, where else would they come from? I mean—who would come in and sneak something into her drawer? And after you explain that four or five times, I go downstairs and take a shower or something. (40 year old niece)

She had a seizure when I moved her on her back. You worry and you think, "That's it. She's not going to make it." I know my father and all, he was crying. You don't know what's happening. When you have a seizure like that you don't know whether she's going to stop breathing and die and you don't know whether she's having a cerebral hemorrhage or what's going on. (35 year old son)

Maintaining patient safety through prevention of falls was a universal and major concern associated with the patient's physical dependence.

The other night I sat him on the foot of the bed and he sat back far enough where he could sit down, but wouldn't you know, I just turned for a minute and he grabbed the footboard and pulled himself right over and he, I mean within a second he just, "zoom," fell. He was upright and then he just did a complete flip in one second. So that's just to give you an idea of what can go wrong and how fast it can go wrong, even though you're doing your best. (26 year old son)

He did fall once, he just kind of went down. It's a good thing we have a good padding on that rug. I saw him laying there and he had the walker on top of him. I thought, "Oh my God, don't tell me that he had a broken hip again." Because he went through two hip operations. I said, "Oh my God, it's

4am, who will I get? Well, maybe I'll have to call the man upstairs." But I said, "Are you hurt? Does anything hurt you?" He said, "No." Well, slowly I pulled him towards the buffet and sort of leaned him against it. Put the walker back on him and gradually picked him up slowly. So from that day on I just watch him. (78 year old wife)

Administration of medications was another area that seemed stressful to family members. Again, it was the mental and physical dependence that necessitated family members taking responsibility for this aspect of care. The number of pills, frequency of administration, and length of time it took some patients to swallow their medications all contributed to difficulties.

It takes 20 minutes to take his pills. That's another thing. I had to shove his pills in his mouth because he refused to take them. One day I called my girlfriend up and said, "He's supposed to take them at 12 and it's 1:30." Not that he would drop dead at 2:00 if he didn't take his pills. It's just that I couldn't get them in. (40 year old wife)

Other areas causing distress for some family members related to bowel and bladder elimination. This was another reminder that patients were no longer able to meet their own basic needs and required assistance from family members.

Thus, family members were forced to alter their interactive patterns to incorporate patients' mental and physical deterioration. Families recognized the need for patience in dealing with their dying relatives. This mental and physical deterioration influenced family members' perceptions of how caring for their dying relatives was "just like having a little baby."

It's just like having a little baby you know, but he's 150 pounds heavier. I take care of a 160 pound baby right now. I've learned to become more patient, all the physical care, the general discipline involved in accepting those not too happy moments of having a baby, you know, middle of the night type of things. I've been dealing with it two years now. (26 year old son)

And I throw things at him. One question after another. "Do you want to get back in bed? Do you want to go brush your teeth? Would you like to stay up for a while and go into another room?" And finally I wasn't getting any response. He was at the point where he wasn't doing much talking anymore. I thought, "Now you've got to stop and sit down and give him time to answer you." So I said, "What do you want me to do Dad?" after I'd thrown out all these things. And it took a long time answering and finally he said, "Be patient." (49 year old daughter)

Interactions with Others

Interactions with others was a second major area of stress for family caregivers. This included maintaining usual family roles and responsibilities, dealing with "well-meaning" family and friends, and personal care aides.

In addition to taking on responsibilities associated with their caregiving roles, most family members needed to maintain their usual responsibilities and eventually, assume their relatives' responsibilities as their conditions deteriorated. At times, some caregivers felt torn between their own nuclear families and caring for their dying relatives. These conflicts centered on trying to keep up with teenagers' busy social activities, needing to leave adolescent children unsupervised while caring for a dying parent hundreds of miles away, and planning a son's wedding.

For some family members it was difficult to deal with the opinions of family and friends who were not directly involved in the caregiving experience. Advice was freely given and often unwanted.

Relatives are starting to push me and tell me that I can't take care of my father. Even one friend that nursed her mother through her final illness said, "Why don't you just put your father in a nursing home and be done with it?" How insensitive of her when she's been through it herself! And this I don't understand. I suppose friends are well meaning, that they are concerned about my life. (49 year old daughter)

For others, family and friends were perceived as insensitive to patients' needs. Discussing the death of others in front of patients or tiring them from prolonged visits were two situations family members found upsetting.

> Two couples came to visit him and then one couple left. The other couple stayed longer and then later on my husband said, "Didn't they think of going home?" That's too much for him. (78 year old wife)

Though personal care aides were employed to help relieve caregivers of some responsibilities, these aides became a source of stress for several families. Aides were not always dependable in terms of showing up at designated times. Thus, family members had to administer difficult care by themselves or were unable to engage in activities outside the home. One primary caregiver employed aides to help with his dying father while he attended college classes. The week before final examinations, the aide quit without notice. One wife hired aides around the clock to help care for her husband. When sickness and car troubles prevented some aides from working, she had to quickly change her work schedule to stay with her husband and seek help from family members to spell her off occasionally. Aides also were suggested as a means of night time relief for a few families who found it impossible to sleep through the night because of constant patient care needs. Unfortunately, having strangers in their homes at night created discomfort and failed to provide the much needed sleep.

> First hospice suggested I should get somebody during the night. So then the first night they sent an aide and it was 3:00 in the morning and I didn't sleep yet because, you know, there's a stranger in the house. (78 year old wife)

Concerns for Self

Concerns for self was the final major area of stress experienced by families. Five areas were identified: putting their lives on hold, personal health, lack of time for themselves, isolation from family and friends, and feelings of guilt.

Many family members found it necessary to put their lives "on hold" once they assumed the caregiving role. Plans were not made, were altered, postponed, or dropped altogether. Major changes in the way they had conducted their lives were necessary to accommodate their new caregiving roles. Two women relocated, one moved 100 miles, the other moved 1500 miles away from family and friends in order to take care of their dying relatives. One son restructured his college courses to accommodate caregiving responsibilities, thus delaying graduation for 18 months. One daughter quit working for a year. This same daughter was unable to make any summer vacation plans with her young family and discouraged her children from entertaining their friends at home because of the bleeding and colostomy odors associated with her mother's cancer. In two families, a non-caregiving family member postponed elective, though major surgery, in order to be more available to the primary caregiver and spare them the added stress of having someone else to worry about.

Personal health concerns began to surface as a source of stress. One young niece experienced exacerbations of her diabetes, rheumatoid arthritis, and peripheral vascular disease, all which she attributed to the stress of caring for her aunt. One caregiver had a degenerative eye condition that destroyed her central vision. Rheumatiod arthritis also affected two elderly wives. In addition, many caregivers commented on how tired they were becoming. A good night's sleep was a rarity.

> I was tired toward the end. I thought I would get sick already. Really, I had lost a lot of weight towards the end. I didn't know what was happening to me because I didn't sleep all night because I was worried about what's going to happen next. It's just a broken record. I'd lay down and I just couldn't fall asleep all night. I was going in circles you know. I wasn't sleeping good and I wasn't eating good either and I was just crying because it was really getting to me. (75 year old wife)

Another consequence of the caregiving role was the absence of time for one's self. The hospice program required that the patient never be left alone, and most of this responsibility was met by the primary caregiver. Though family members and friends were help-ful with errands, primary caregivers felt a strong need for some "alone time," time for themselves, free from caregiving responsi-bilities, to do whatever they wanted.

> I think the biggest problem I have is I really don't have anywhere to go. There's no alone time at all. There's just no where to go. It's just gotten so bad here. (40 year old niece)

> I get more stir crazy when you just can't get out or when you have to stay completely on tap. It's like you don't move out of this area. I'd have to wait for somebody to be home to even go and take a shower. But with last week when he was having one problem after another, you didn't want to be even that far away. (49 year old wife)

For the two women who moved from their own homes to care for their dying relatives, feelings of isolation from family and friends were an added stress. This separation was difficult and, at various times throughout the caregiving experience, both women expressed the desire to be home to the degree that alternative caregiving ar-rangements were being considered. Absence of their normal rou-tines within their normal social and physical environment seemed the basis of this stress.

Guilt was a final source of stress related to caregivers' concerns for self. Though feelings of guilt seemed no more stressful than previously discussed areas, circumstances associated with guilt were numerous and at times, complex. Figure 1 displays the link-ages involved in caregivers' expressions of guilt.

Four circumstances lead to the expression of guilt: (a) wanting the caregiving experience to be over, (b) not spending enough time with their dying relatives, (c) being less vigilant about caregiving responsibilities, and (d) being impatient with and insensitive to their relatives. In each of these four circumstances, family members were unable to fulfill self-expectations of how they should behave toward and feel about their dying relatives. Families seemed to have established ideas that defined appropriate interaction patterns with their dying relatives. Consequently, if they did not live up to their self-expectations, they felt guilty.

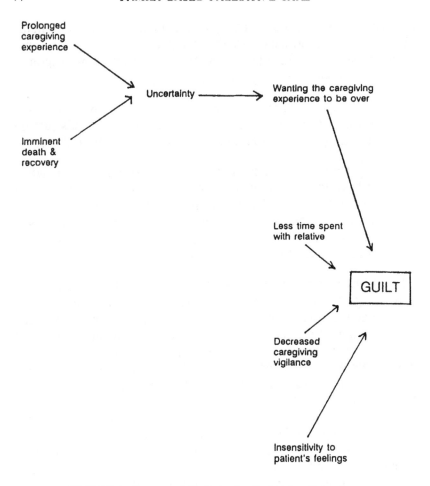

FIGURE 1. Sources of Guilt in the Caregiving Experience

Two situations seemed to precede families' wishes for the care-giving experience to be over. Some families experienced caregiving responsibilities that extended beyond their expectations. Families entered the hospice program thinking that their caregiving role would involve a short term commitment, most often less than 6 or 7 months. When patients lived beyond their medical prognoses, and beyond the expectations families had regarding the need to maintain their caregiving roles, serious problems arose. Families began to question when their caregiving experiences would be over, and then felt guilty about their needs to end this role because they realized the end would occur when their relatives died.

> I was going to make her last days, months, weeks, whatever, the best that I could, but then as it goes on, it's like, I'm getting tired of doing this. And it's not that I love her any less. I'm sure that when she and I know that it, that eventually she'll get bad again, I'll probably feel the same as I did in the beginning, but it's the in between time that I don't want to do this anymore. (40 year old daughter)

> This is ridiculous. Nine months of having a veg (vegetable), somebody that's not your husband. It's just going on so long. I told a friend, "I've got a light at the end of my tunnel," but I'm beginning to think now that there's no light. For a while there when he just wasn't getting worse and the CATT scan showed his tumor hadn't grown, I thought that this is never going to be over. I don't remember what life was like. All I know is that the other day I cried myself to sleep thinking, "This is what I'm going to remember!" If it had ended five months ago I think I would have had nice memories, but now, I don't wish him to die, I wish my life was in order. I'm stagnant. I'm in limbo. I'm not here. I'm not there. (40 year old wife)

Other families were faced with their relatives' unexpected recoveries after preparing for an imminent death. When families were told, often on several occasions, that their relatives would die within a few days, they prepared themselves for the imminent death, alerted others to the situation, and said their goodbyes. When these patients unexpectedly recovered, families had great difficulty readjusting their attitudes and feelings to focus again on the patient and their own responsibilities as caregivers. Their energy had been used to prepare themselves for their relatives' deaths, and when their conditions improved, there was little energy left to revert back to the caregiving situation.

Even though my mother was in the program only a short time, when we thought she was going to die she was in the hospice free-standing unit. And then she was coming back home again and that was a rollercoaster kind of feeling because you feel she's gone, she's going to die, and then she comes home and first you're happy she's gone and she's going to die and you're not going to have any worries, and then all of a sudden she's coming home and you're looking forward to having her come home. And then the staff called and said that she's not doing too good and she won't come home today, she'll come home tomorrow. You're always up and down. If I had six months of this I'd need a support group! (64 year old daughter)

Inherent in the situation of prolonged caregiving as well as the experience of imminent death and recovery, was a great deal of uncertainty that, in itself, was stressful for families. The caregiving role within the structure of a terminal cancer illness was a new situation for all families. This was an unfamiliar event for which they had little previous experience or knowledge about how this situation would evolve. The absence of a definite time frame as a reference for the end of their caregiving situations often led to negative and frightening feelings.

The only thing is, and they (the hospice staff) can't do anything about it, is not knowing. Even though when we get to where we feel like we need some kind of answers and we need something, in the back of your mind you're wondering if there's something new happening, if there's something different going on. There's the uncertainty. We don't know. She looks good but we don't know what could happen tonight or tomorrow. (40 year old daughter)

The uncertainty resulting from perceptions of prolonged caregiving and the cycle of imminent death and recovery ultimately lead family members to question their relatives' prognoses and wish that the end were near.

> I'm sure they're all (the hospice staff) sick and tired of me whining, "When is it going to be over?" You know it sounds mercenary, I know it sounds mercenary, but I'm not going to have any guilt feelings about it because, you know (the saying), "Walk a mile in my shoes. . . ." I have guilts wanting him alive, wanting my kids to have a father, wanting to have a husband, wanting my mother-in-law to have a child, but yet, I wish it was over already. Living with guilt feelings, you know, selfishly for myself. I want it all over, but having guilt feelings because he's still enjoying life, what there is of it. (40 year old wife)

Thus, one source of guilt was derived from a pattern of circumstances set in motion by situations of prolonged caregiving, imminent death and unexpected recovery, followed by uncertainty and the wish that this part of their lives was over.

Guilt was expressed again when families felt they were not spending enough time with their dying relatives. Families felt they should be with the patients more during the home care experience and also felt bad when they utilized the respite unit. Even though they realized there had to be limits on time with their relatives because of other responsibilities, nevertheless they continued to feel guilty for not meeting their self-expectations.

> I just want her to know that I'm here as much as I can. A lot of times it's hard. That's important to me because I do feel a lot of, a certain amount of guilt which I shouldn't feel because I can't help that I live eight hours away, but I wish I could be in two places at once. (37 year old daughter)

> And I just get these real guilt feelings about putting him in FSU, but you know, he likes it. I feel I'm only going there (FSU) because I feel I should be with him. There's a lot of guilt. But let's face it, I didn't spend 24 hours a day with him when he was well, how can I start now? (40 year old wife)

Families took pride in their caregiving abilities and felt a great deal of responsibility for the patients' well being. Guilt was expressed in the instances where family members felt they were less vigilant than they should have been and, thus, caused unnecessary discomfort for their relatives. This was especially true for one woman whose husband was immobile, unable to communicate, and therefore, totally dependent on others for all his needs.

> Urine was coming both ways (through the urinary catheter and leaking around the catheter). I gave him his medicines at 7:30 and turned him at 8. At 10 I went to feed him and the whole bed was soaked and yet it was still coming through the tube. And I felt like a big heel, but yet how would you know it, or even check under the covers for that short period of time? But you feel like a heel when here's all the sheet wet, like you're being neglectful. (49 year old wife)

Other feelings of guilt occurred when family members were impatient with their relatives and insensitive to their feelings. Families no longer felt comfortable if they displayed anger. It was as if the old patterns of interaction were no longer appropriate now that their relatives were dying. Interestingly, feelings of guilt occurred *during* the caregiving experience, while denial of guilty feelings occurred *after* their relatives' deaths. It may be that when family members focused on the day-to-day caregiving experience, details of their interactions with their relatives were more vivid, so perceived transgressions against them were still fresh in their minds and more easily recalled. In contrast, after their relatives' deaths, reference points and orientations seemed to change. Family members became less concerned with their day-to-day interactions with their relatives, and now evaluated their performance based on the entire caregiving experience as a whole. Thus, when they reflected back and summarized their behaviors, family members were far less critical of themselves and far more satisfied with their overall performance as caregivers.

DISCUSSION

Families were very open about sharing the difficult parts of their caregiving experiences. Though questions addressing this area were part of the interview guide used during the first visit, families often volunteered this information as they reviewed the history of their relatives' cancer and what caring for them had been like so far. Thus, direct questions frequently were unnecessary. In addition, families discussed the stresses they were confronted with in a calm and matter of fact manner. Typically, they did not seem to be complaining, but just recounting difficult situations. When the investigator commented on how difficult caring for their dying relatives seemed, families minimized the seriousness of their stresses and tended to be very accepting of these problems as part of the responsibilities they willingly assumed. Though specific circumstances were upsetting when they occurred, families seemed able to move quickly beyond stressful incidents and continue with caregiving.

Sources of caregiver stress that emerged from this study are well documented throughout the literature, especially those associated with caring for a cognitively impaired relative (Barusch, 1988; Chenoweth & Spencer, 1986; Moritz, Kasl, & Berkman, 1989; Motenko, 1989; Romeis, 1989; Stetz, 1989; Zarit, Reever, & Bach-Peterson, 1980). Though families seemed able to incorporate most stresses into their caregiving routines, changes in their relatives' mental status created problems that were more constant and more difficult to deal with. The reciprocal nature of families' relationships with their relatives was noticeably absent. Often families could no longer derive support, understanding, or previous role responsibilities from their dying relatives. Even basic communication was limited or nonexistent. Memories could not be shared and some families felt they were caring for a stranger. Barusch (1988) found that missing the relationship that had been established over many years was the most common problem identified by elderly spouse caregivers. Beyond this sense of loss, for several hospice families it was as if their relatives were already dead. At times this loss seemed to make it difficult to maintain the caregiving role. Their tolerance diminished, they became more fatigued and they began to wish for "the end."

Several women caregivers in this study seemed caught between two generations, simultaneously caring for their children and a dying parent (Brody, 1981; Miller, 1981). Even those who were caring for a dying spouse rather than a dying parent still had caregiving responsibilities to their aging parents and thus were caring for three generations of their families. Feelings of isolation, loss of personal time, and putting their lives on hold were common themes discussed by caregivers in this study. Other researchers have identified similar stresses (Cantor, 1983; Hasselkus, 1988; Holing, 1986). Neugarten (1977) refers to the "off-time" event of the caregiving experience, especially for the middle-aged women caregivers. The unexpectedness of assuming total care of their dying spouses or parents had not been in their overall plan for that time. Once they became caregivers, priorities had to shift and personal, family, and professional plans had to change.

In contrast to the caregiving literature, concerns about pain, financial worries, and interactions with professional staff were not identified as sources of stress for families in this study. Several explanations seem relevant. In regard to pain, the hospice philosophy of pain control involves analgesic administration on a continual, around the clock schedule, rather than the more traditional "as necessary" use. Therefore any new pain or any previous pain that was no longer helped by the current analgesic regimen was usually controlled within 12-24 hours and did not present a major problem. The cost of care was not an issue because the particular hospice from which caregivers were drawn assumed responsibility for any costs that were not covered by insurance. Also it was during this time that the 210 day limit on hospice services covered by Medicare benefits was removed. Hospice Medicare benefits were in effect until the patients' deaths.

The lack of tension resulting from caregivers' interactions with the professional hospice staff involves a more tentative explanation. It is suggested that the palliative goals of hospice care were shared openly by families and hospice staff and as such, contributed to a common purpose. All knew and accepted the patients' terminal diagnoses. This knowledge minimized discordant expectations regarding treatment options and nursing care interventions. In addition, this particular hospice conducted an extensive pre-employment interview that encouraged potential employees to share their reasons for choosing hospice care and their feelings about death and working with dying patients and their families. This may lead to a more committed and actively involved staff who genuinely value what they are doing and respect patients' and families' desires to control the final days. Also it is suggested that hospice staff may have a similarity in experience with caregiving families that is not found in non-hospice situations. That is, more hospice staff may have experienced the death of a loved one and therefore, are better able to empathize with families caring for dying relatives. It may be that within non-hospice caregiving situations staff have not yet experienced caring for frail or elderly family members and therefore have not yet considered how they would perceive that experience as a family caregiver.

Findings from this study have been examined from within the larger body of research on caregivers. However, several characteristics of hospice care distinguish it from the non-hospice caregiving situations that were the focus of other caregiver investigations. First, length of the caregiving experience was typically much shorter for hospice families, often less than 6 months. Non-hospice family caregivers frequently had spent up to 5 to 10 years or longer caring for their relatives. Second, hospice patients and their families knew the terminal nature of their diagnoses. Thus, the stress associated with protective caregiving (Bower, 1987), i.e., devising elaborate schemes to protect their relatives from knowledge of their deteriorating conditions, were not necessary. Finally, the age of the hospice caregivers was younger than non-hospice caregivers. Many studies investigated elderly caregivers. Therefore, the comparisons made should be viewed as tentative at this time.

Though this article focused on stresses families encountered as they cared for their dying relatives at home, families did manage to confront the difficulties of their caregiving roles and cope effectively. Techniques used to manage the identified stresses will be described in a future article. In addition, families discussed positive aspects of caregiving and their decisions to assume this responsibility for their dying relatives. Several factors were central to families' motivations for entering and maintaining the caregiving role. These included ensuring personhood, maintaining control, belonging, and maintaining attachment. The interplay of these factors and how they were manifested within hospice caregiving experiences also will be the focus of a future article.

PRACTICE IMPLICATIONS AND FUTURE RESEARCH

Allowing families to identify sources of stress from their own life situations and points of view as hospice caregivers enhances our understanding of what home care of relatives dying from cancer is like. Several areas of concern seem amenable to interventions by health care professionals. First, when mental deterioration begins to interfere with patients' abilities to continue functioning in supportive and reciprocal roles, health care professionals can assist caregiving families in developing alternative sources of support. Open discussions about the impact of changes in their relatives' mental status, what to expect, and how to react effectively may help families prepare for these difficulties and ultimately find them less stressful. The concern for the prevention of falls was expressed by all families and seems to be an area where teaching of basic safety precautions could enable families to accurately assess their relatives' needs for supervision in this area.

Identified stresses involved areas other than direct caregiving, consistent with Bower's (1987) reconceptualization of caregiving. Families need to be encouraged to take care of themselves both physically and emotionally. Health professionals can assist families by getting them to accept offers of help, set limits on the demands of their caregiving roles, and take time to enjoy other areas of their lives. Helping families examine realistic self-expectations could minimize feelings of guilt and allow a healthier, more positive perception of their value as caregivers.

Future research needs to explore further the meaning families attach to their relatives' deterioration in mental status and ways to cope more effectively with this problem. Closer and more extensive examination of the resources and coping abilities of families whose relatives experience this deterioration and families whose relatives maintain intact mental function is warranted. Elderly caregivers in this study seemed to describe stresses less frequently and with less intensity. Reanalysis of data by age may uncover differences in attitudes or purposes that would enhance understanding of this experience for different generations. Additional areas to compare further include families with very young children versus families with grown children. The observation that hospice nurses were not a source of stress needs to be pursued. What was the role of the hospice nurses? How were they perceived by family caregivers? What are their interventions like and are they different from those in non-hospice caregiving situations? Extending data collection to include the first year after their relatives' deaths would enable various outcome measures to be assessed for all phenomena.

Within the hospice philosophy, health care professionals have long addressed the family as the unit of care and are in a unique position to assist families as they care for dying relatives at home. Continuing to focus research on caregiving families has the potential for generating new knowledge about how hospice professionals can most effectively support families through one of life's most difficult experiences.

REFERENCES

Barusch, A. S. (1988). Problems and coping strategies of elderly spouse caregivers. *The Gerontologist, 28,* 677-685.

Bower, B. J. (1987). Intergenerational caregiving: Adult caregivers and their aging parents. *Advances in Nursing Science, 9*(2), 20-31.

Brody, E. (1981). Women in the middle and family help to older people. *Gerontologist, 21,* 471-480.

Cantor, M. H. (1983). Strain among caregivers: A study of experience in the United States. *The Gerontologist, 23,* 597-604.

Chenoweth, B., & Spencer, B. (1986). Dementia: the experience of family caregivers. *The Gerontologist, 26,* 267-272.

Corbin, J. (1986). Qualitative data analysis for grounded theory. In W.C. Chenitz & J.M. Swanson (Eds.), *From practice to grounded theory: Qualitative research in nursing* (pp. 102-120). Menlo Park, CA: Addison Wesley.

Garland, T.N., Bass, D.M., & Otto, M.E. (1984). The needs of hospice patients and primary caregivers: A comparison of primary caregivers' and hospice nurses' perceptions. *American Journal of Hospice Care, 1*(3), 40-45.

Glaser, B.G. (1978). *Theoretical sensitivity.* Mill Valley, CA: The Sociology Press.

Glaser, B.G., & Strauss, A.L. (1967). *The discovery of grounded theory: Strategies for qualitative research.* New York: Aldine.

Googe, M.C., & Varricchio, C.G. (1981). A pilot investigation of home health care needs of cancer patients and their families. *Oncology Nursing Forum, 8,* 24-29.

Grobe, M.E., Ilstrup, D.M., & Ahmann, D.L. (1981). Skills needed by family members to maintain the care of an advanced cancer patient. *Cancer Nursing, 4,* 371-375.

Guba, E.G., & Lincoln, Y.S. (1981). *Effective evaluation.* San Francisco: Jossey-Bass.

Hasselkus, B. R. (1988). Meaning in family caregiving: Perspectives on caregiver/professional relationships. *The Gerontologist, 28,* 686-691.

Hinds, C. (1985). The needs of families who care for patients with cancer at home: Are we meeting them? *Journal of Advanced Nursing, 10,* 575-581.

Holing, E. V. (1986). The primary caregiver's perception of the dying trajectory. *Cancer Nursing, 9,* 29-37.

McGinnis, S. S. (1986). How can nurses improve the quality of life of the hospice client and family?: An exploratory study. *The Hospice Journal, 2*(1), 23-36.

Miller, D. A. (1981). The sandwich generation, adult children of the aging. *Social Work, 26,* 419-423.

Moritz, D. J., Kasl, S. V., & Berkman, L. F. (1989). The health impact of living with a cognitively impaired elderly spouse: Depression symptoms and social functioning. *Journal of Gerontology, 44*(1), 17-27.

Motenko, A. K. (1989). The frustrations, gratifications, and well-being of dementia caregivers. *The Gerontologist, 29,* 166-172.

National Hospice Organization. (1988). *A guide to the nation's hospices.* Arlington, VA: Author.

Neugarten, B. L. (1977). Personality and aging. In J. E. Birren & K. W. Schaie (Eds.), *Handbook of the psychology of aging.* New York: Van Nostrand Reinhold.

Romeis, J. C. (1989). Caregiver strain: Toward an enlarged perspective. *Journal of Aging and Health, 1*(2), 188-208.

Sandelowski, M. (1986). The problem of rigor in qualitative research. *Advances in Nursing Science, 8*(3), 27-37.

Skorupka, P., & Bohnet, N. (1982). Primary caregivers' perceptions of nursing behavior that best meet their needs in a home care hospice setting. *Cancer Nursing, 5,* 371-374.

Stetz, K. M. (1989). The relationship among background characteristics, purpose in life and caregiving demands on perceived health of spouse caregivers. *Scholarly Inquiry for Nursing Practice: An International Journal, 3*(2), 133-153.

Zarit, S. H., Reever, K. E., & Bach-Peterson, J. (1980). Relatives of the impaired elderly: Correlates of feelings of burden. *The Gerontologist, 20,* 649-655.

The Work of Patients and Spouses in Managing Advanced Cancer at Home

Nola Martens

Betty Davies

SUMMARY. The purpose of this paper is to report the findings of a descriptive study which identified the resources used by patients with advanced cancer and their spouses to manage at home. Data were collected through semi-structured interviews with a sample of seven couples identified through two ambulatory clinics at a regional cancer institute. Participants were patients with advanced cancer, between the ages of 45 and 66, and their spouses. Interviews, conducted with each individual and with each couple, were audiotaped, transcribed, and subjected to qualitative analysis. Content analysis showed that patients and spouses utilized internal and external resources, and that external resources were either physical or interpersonal in nature. Conceptual analysis indicated that both patients and spouses dealt with facing either inevitable or uncertain death by engaging in various types of "work." Understanding the dimensions of such work has implications for health care professionals caring for patients and families in palliative care.

The stressful nature of the family's experience when a member has advanced cancer has been well documented in both lay and

---

Nola Martens, RN, MN, has been clinically involved with patients with cancer, and their families, for several years. She is Education Consultant in oncology nursing, and Research Associate for a research project focusing on families in supportive care. Betty Davies, RN, PhD, has been involved in the areas of terminal care and bereavement for many years. Most recently, she has been conducting research in these areas, focusing specifically on the experience of children following the death of a sibling and of families in supportive care. She is Associate Professor with the School of Nursing, University of British Columbia, and holds an Investigatorship Award with the Research Division, British Columbia Children's Hospital. Address correspondence to Dr. Davies at The School of Nursing, U.B.C., T.206-2211 Wesbrook Mall, Vancouver, B.C., Canada V6T 2B5.

Acknowledgement is given to the Alberta Foundation for Nursing Research for partial funding of this research.

professional health care literature. With very few exceptions, health care writers begin their discussion with the acknowledgement that cancer is the most feared of all diseases which carries with it a sense of impending death, stigma, and isolation for the individual with the disease. Within a family systems perspective, it is well known that illness in one member of a family unit has a major impact on all family members. Furthermore, families are expected to assume more care of their loved one with advanced cancer in the home for as long as possible and to the point of death, if that is feasible. These facts — the stressful nature of cancer, the diffuse effects of cancer on the entire family, and the growing expectation that care will be provided in the home for as long as possible — require a clear understanding by health care professionals of what care at home requires of families, and of what families require in order to manage. To this end, it is important that professionals not only deal with the traumatic effects of the disease itself, but also identify the strengths and resources of the patient and family managing advanced cancer in the home, and understand this situation from the perspective of those directly involved. The purposes of this paper therefore are (1) to describe the resources identified by patients with advanced cancer and their spouses as useful in their managing home care; and (2) to describe a conceptualization of resource use as "work."

REVIEW OF LITERATURE

When cancer is experienced in one of the partners, the effects on the marital subsystem are particularly difficult. In one study, widows of cancer patients suffered more stress during the terminal phase than in widowhood, and they had more difficulty than widows whose husbands died of cardiac disease (Vachon et al., 1977). In addition, older spouses may experience decline in health and strength due to the demands of home care; therefore, support to these caregivers is of concern to health care providers. The older age group within the population is increasing; cancer is a disease which affects older more than younger age groups. In 1986, 80% of people with cancer were between the ages of 55 to 65 plus (*Canadian Cancer Statistics*, 1988). Therefore, home care for people with cancer will become even more important than it is at present, and any improvement in the understanding of what couples experience in managing at home will be vital.

Researchers report that the spouse is often responsible for the majority of home care (Creek, 1982; Gotay, 1984; Zajac, 1985). Furthermore, the obligation to provide care leads to restricted social contacts for the family caregiver (Cassileth & Hamilton, 1979; Gotay, 1984). In fact, when just the patient and spouse live together, they are less likely to receive help from friends and neighbors than are those who live with other family members or friends (Cartwright, Hockey, & Anderson, 1973). In a study of home care for 44 patients, Pringle and Taylor (1984) reported that 40% received care only from the spouses without help from anyone else. While the family's experience of providing home care to a child has been described (Martinson et al., 1986), the experience of providing home care to an older adult has not received much attention although considerable work has been done on caregivers for frail older persons. Furthermore, concurrent examination of both patients and spouses has been done in relatively few studies, and then only related to specific concerns about types of nursing interventions (Freihofer & Felton, 1976). In one major study conducted in the United States, both patients and their primary care providers were assessed using various objective measures to examine costs and other selected outcomes (Mor, Greer, & Kastenbaum, 1988). This assessment however did not focus specifically on the experience of the couple in managing their situation. The majority of studies are retrospective, occurring after the patient's death. Some conclusions are derived solely from chart reviews which document patient services rendered (Gotay, 1984; Zajac, 1985). To overcome these perceived deficits in published studies, the focus of the present study was the marital dyad in which one member has advanced cancer and is at home.

METHODS

In order to understand the perspective of the individuals (patients and spouses) directly involved with the palliative care situation, a qualitative study of several couples was conducted. The purpose of qualitative research is to "gain a fuller understanding of what constitutes reality for the participants in a particular real-life setting" (Field & Morse, 1985, p. 111). In this approach, validity is strengthened by deliberate techniques which ground the data in the experience of the subjects, rather than in the perspective of the researcher (LeCompte & Goetz, 1982), and by the method's emphasis upon the richness or depth of data, rather than its breadth. This means that instead of the traditional reliance upon numerical analyses of selected objective characteristics of a large sample, in-depth investigations of the subjective experience of a relatively small number of knowledgeable subjects are used. Since the purpose of qualitative research is to understand or describe a poorly understood phenomenon from the perspective of the person experiencing the phenomenon, to conceptualize the phenomenon, and eventually to develop theory which can then be tested in future research, no attempt is made to control for extraneous variables or to place experimental controls on the phenomenon.

Sample

Subjects were recruited from the outpatient clinic of a regional cancer institute in Western Canada. Criteria for participation were that the patients were over 45 years of age; had their spouse as primary caregiver; were able to read and write English; and were judged by the clinic staff not to be significantly burdened by participation in the study. In addition, both patients and their spouses had to give informed consent. Initially, potential subjects were identified from a clinic which served clients requiring symptom management during the final stages of illness. Because recruitment progressed slowly, due to the available patients not meeting the criteria, a second clinic was used for subject recruitment. This clinic included patients in a somewhat earlier phase of palliative care.

From both clinics, 13 patients were identified who met the criteria; of these, 7 patients and their spouses agreed to participate. Reasons for not participating were: 1 male patient did not wish to discuss his case; another male patient felt it would be of no help to him; 3 female patients agreed but their spouses declined; and, 1 couple agreed but a mutually acceptable time could not be agreed upon. All seven patients in the study had metastatic cancer resulting from primary sites in the colon, head and neck, liver, or stomach. The time since diagnosis ranged from 4 years to 3 months before data collection. Of the 7 patients, 3 were male and 4 female, ranging in age from 46 to 66 years, with an average age of 55 years. Age of spouses ranged from 44 to 68, with an average age of 53 years. All participants were Caucasian.

Data Collection

Qualitative research methods of taped interviews, observations recorded in field notes, and diary notations were used to collect data. A semi-structured interview guide was developed based on a literature review and suggestions from subject experts, and was tested for clarity and effectiveness with three couples who met the study criteria. The interview guide* consisted of open-ended questions pertaining to the physical, emotional, and spiritual resources the couples used to manage, the effect of the disease on their life, and how they were managing. Interviews were conducted in the couples' homes at times convenient to them. Each member of the couple was interviewed twice alone. Second interviews, usually much shorter than the first, were used to clarify any statements from the first interview which were ambiguous. A portion of the final interview was conducted with both members of each couple to clarify preceding data as necessary, to ask questions about the effect of participating in the study, and to elicit suggestions for health care professionals. Each interview, ranging from 45 minutes to 2 hours in length, was audiotaped and transcribed to ensure accurate representation of what each individual said.

Data Analysis

Interviews were recorded, transcribed and subjected to qualitative analysis. Content analysis identified types and sources of resources each couple used. In addition, the transcripts, field notes, and diary notations were analyzed for recurrent patterns, categories,

---

*A copy of the interview guide is available upon request from the authors.

and themes and for emergent concepts using comparative analytic techniques for qualitative data (Glaser, 1978; Glaser & Strauss, 1967). Transcripts were read line by line, identifying words, or codes, that captured the meaning of the lines. In addition, each transcript was reviewed for similarities and differences. Codes were compared with one another within the same transcript, with codes within other transcripts, and entire transcripts were compared with one another. "Theoretical saturation" was achieved when certain categories consistently emerged and little new information was discovered (Glaser, 1978).

This process facilitated the generation of a theoretical framework which describes and explains the work of managing advanced cancer at home. Assumptions underlying this method are those of naturalistic or emic research, in which the participants' view of reality, represented by their perceptions and descriptions of the world, are regarded as the reality that affects subsequent behavior (May, 1982). To enhance validity, selected interviews were read by an expert in qualitative analysis, and the categories, themes, and conceptualization were examined. In addition, the themes and categories were reviewed with the seventh couple in order to ensure accurate representation of the participants' views.

RESULTS

Resources Used

Both patients and spouses identified resources, classified as internal and external, that were of aid to them in their supportive care experience. Internal resources for patients were those strengths, traits or behaviors which came from within the patient, such as their own character or faith, originating from their childhood, background or past death-related experiences. Internal resources also included activities or mental processes patients utilized to manage their situation. Patients' external resources were either physical or interpersonal. Physical resources were medications and information dealing with diagnosis, prognosis, and treatment. Professionals were the source of physical resources; family and friends were the source of interpersonal resources in the form of care, comfort, love and interest. Care included preparing special foods and reminding to take medications. Comfort involved the provision of a nice environment, "encouragement when I'm down," and being listened to. Interest was evident to patients when family members were involved and when they provided distractions through family activities.

The majority of the resources used by the patients with advanced cancer came from within themselves and from their families, in particular from their spouses. Patients wanted a professional available to answer questions and to provide the facts in a way that was understandable and compassionate. Clinic staff were viewed as the source of obtaining medications to control disease or treatment related symptoms, such as pain, nausea, or constipation. It was the family's role however to listen, support, care, and provide expressions of love.

For spouses, their identified resources were not specific to themselves, but were relevant only as they required help to care for the patient. They too identified internal resources, such as faith, attitude, and keeping busy. They, however, did not delve into their own character strengths or engage in self-reflection as the patients did. For spouses, external resources from professionals came mainly in the form of disease-related information. Interpersonal resources for spouses centered mainly around talking and having relationships with others. The patients, friends, and children were the sources of interpersonal help. Thus, the critical role that family members play for each other in managing situations of supportive care was emphasized by both the patients and spouses.

Uncertainty/Inevitability of Death

All patients had advanced cancer which had the potential of ending their lives in the near future. Within the total group, however, two groups of patients were identified according to their view of the inevitability of their death. The first group (N = 3) talked about their death as inevitable. They were no longer receiving any treatment, they had been told by their physician that their disease was terminal, and they had physical symptoms such as pain, weight loss and immobility. The second group (N = 4), although realizing the potential for death existed, did not perceive death as an immediate threat. They were still receiving some form of treatment, even if only for palliation, or desired further treatment; they were not experiencing physical symptoms, or had symptoms but denied the need for interventions because their day-to-day life was not physically impeded. Patients' perceptions of death as uncertain or inevitable changed as their condition worsened, and patients with these differing perceptions went about their work in different ways.

Spouses did not divide into two groups as patients did according to any characteristic unique to themselves although they too faced slightly different tasks, depending on patient group. For all spouses however, death was described as uncertain, even when the patients perceived their own death as inevitable. For spouses to admit that the patients' death was inevitable communicated a sense of giving up, and for the spouses, it was important for patients' wellbeing to appear optimistic about the eventual outcome.

Work of Patients and Spouses

It was clear from the constant comparative analysis that all respondents, in dealing with advanced cancer at home, had "work" to do. Both patients and spouses engaged in several types of work to manage the situation of advanced cancer. Each type had a goal and a focus, and required the investment of energy and resources for the goals to be accomplished. The focus of the work differed for patients and spouses. Patients' work focused mainly on themselves; spouses' work focused mainly on the patients. Patients focused primarily on what they personally had to do to face the inevitability or uncertainty of their death. Spouses, within the boundaries of their own strengths and weaknesses, focused their work on doing what was best for the patient. They applied their energies to the task of caring for their ill husband or wife for an undetermined length of time, facing an outcome that had a varying degree of uncertainty attached to it.

One type of work, hoping, applied to both patients and spouses and serves to illustrate the different foci. For both patients and spouses, the goal was to achieve an optimal or desirable outcome. For patients who saw death as uncertain the goal was disease-related outcomes, such as cure; for those who saw their death as inevitable, they sought comfort-related outcomes, such as a pain-free afternoon. The focus was themselves. For spouses, the goal was also for a desirable outcome, not for oneself but for the patient. When the patient viewed death as uncertain, the spouse hoped in a global way for the patient's cure; when the patient viewed death as inevitable, the spouse hoped specifically for the patient's comfort.

Hoping was the only type of work common to both patients and spouses; the other categories of work were different for patients and spouses although the types of work complemented each other. Patients worked at hoping, controlling, preparing, maintaining, daily living, and fighting. Spouses worked at surviving, preserving, taking stock, and helping. A summary of the types of patient work, indicating the goal and focus for each type is provided in Table 1. The same information pertaining to spouses' work is presented in Table 2.

Controlling and Surviving

The overwhelming psychological effect of the disease on both patients and spouses led to one dominant category of work for both groups. For patients, controlling predominated; for spouses, surviving was dominant. For patients, the goal of controlling was to control aspects of self in response to the physical and emotional strain of having a cancer diagnosis. Patients in the uncertain group worked at regaining control of their physical bodies in order to work toward being healthier. Patients in the inevitable group, however, recognized that there were limits to how much control they could have over their bodies, and instead focussed on careful management of their time and energy.

The goal of spouse surviving was to "carry on" or "hang on" during the periods of either relative disease stability or disease progression in the patients' life. Spouses of patients in the uncertain group were concerned with managing the intellectual awareness of the outcome. For spouses whose husband or wife was a member of the inevitable group, the focus was on managing the progressive physical decline of the patient. For all spouses, surviving included keeping their minds occupied with other things and keeping physically busy with day-to-day activities such as maintaining a job, shopping, or keeping house.

Table 1
Types of Patient Work

Type	Goal	Focus by Patient Group	
		Death: Uncertain	Death: Inevitable
1. Hoping	To achieve an optimal/ desirable outcome.	Seeking disease-related outcomes.	Seeking comfort related outcomes.
2. Controlling	To control self in the situation.	Utilizing physical and mental processes to manage thoughts: use of mind to heal body.	Utilizing physical and mental processes to manage thoughts: recognition of limitations and concerns for energy conservation.
3. Preparing	To plan ahead in order to equip the family to manage following the patient's death.	Worrying and thinking about the future.	Carrying out explicit and concrete actions for the future.
4. Maintaining	To maintain the support from others and to help others deal with the situation.	Recognizing the importance of their attitudes on the family's support and ability to manage.	Recognizing the importance of their attitudes on the family's support and ability to manage.
5. Daily Living	To go on living a meaningful life in spite of cancer.	Outlining generalities of normal life.	Outlining specifics of how they manage.
6. Fighting	To do the best they could against the disease.	Looking ahead to a war. Preparing to engage in a fight.	Engaging in specific battles, meeting specific goals; they acknowledge they will lose but that they will fight.

Table 2
Types of Spouse Work

Type	Goal	Focus by Patient Group	
		Death: Uncertain	Death: Inevitable
1. Hoping	To have a desirable outcome for the patient.	On global hopes for cure or a miracle.	On specific hopes for patient comfort, short term goal attainment and spiritual re-unity.
2. Surviving	To protect and care for the patient and family.	On giving mainly psychological support, being positive.	On giving physical as well as psychological support, maintaining a role for the patient.
3. Preserving	To "hang on" or "carry on" during the situation.	On managing the strain of uncertainty in disease outcome in their loved one's illness.	On managing the strain of watching their loved one's progressive illness.
4. Taking Stock	To assess the pre-illness life with the patient.	On reviewing the patient's character and their shared experiences.	On reviewing the patient's character and their shared experiences.

Preparing and Taking Stock

The work of both patients and spouses involved an element of preparing for possible or certain patient death. For patients, this involved preparing; for spouses, it involved the work of taking stock. Patients in the uncertain group thought and worried about the future within a perceived ambiguous context. In contrast, patients in the inevitable group described concrete behaviors and well thought out strategies as they prepared their families and themselves for death. These concrete behaviors included completion of wills, funeral plans, and lists of what to do around the house. For patients in both groups, it was important to receive information from health care professionals and then to give this information to the families in a manner acceptable both to the patient's style and the family's needs.

All spouses prepared for the loss of their loved one through a process of taking stock of their shared life and their loved one's character. Taking stock involved the discussion of their past life together, where they lived, and how they related, including the enjoyments and struggles of their marriage. Important to this work was the relationship with the patient, the spouse's mental process of reliving their shared life, and talking about the patient to others.

Maintaining and Preserving

One category of work for both patients and spouses involved an attempt to manage the intangibles of family life within the context of advanced cancer. For patients, it was important to maintain regular family life, both for their own sake and for the sake of their loved ones. As one patient said, "I will not allow the cancer to eat away at the very fabric of the home." Patients realized that their families required a strong will and sufficient energy levels to keep going, and provided for this through maintaining a positive attitude which served two purposes: it made it "easier for people to be around," and it kept "despair from afflicting others."

Spouses engaged in preserving work to keep the family and its memories intact. Spouses of patients in the uncertain group concentrated on creating memories, enjoying family life with the patient, and changing their priorities. Spouses of patients in the inevitable group concentrated on reviewing memories, healing past hurts, and making the best of the time left.

Daily Living and Helping

Patients' daily living work was complemented by spouses' helping work. Daily living work included those tasks which allowed patients to maintain as normal a life as possible. Activities of daily living took on more importance as patients realized the inevitability of their death. The accomplishment of simple household tasks helped them deal with their illness by allowing them to feel useful and productive. Spouses' helping work included being supportive to patients through monitoring and meeting the patients' physical needs for such things as food and rest, and watching for psychological reactions such as depression or giving up. Spouses of patients in the inevitable group were also concerned with maintaining a role for the patients and providing an atmosphere where the patients could function as normally as possible.

Fighting and Helping

Patients worked directly at fighting the disease; spouses were only able to fight indirectly by helping the patients with their fight. Spouses did not work at fighting; instead their helping work complemented the patients' fighting work. The goal of fighting was for patients to do the best they could against their disease. Both groups of patients discussed "fighting" the situation. However, the descriptions of fighting by patients in the uncertain group lacked detail: "As long as I still have my two feet and my head's still working, I'm still fighting it, I guess." In contrast, a quote from a patient in the inevitable group illustrates the detailed mental image of his fight:

> Battling an illness and battling cancer is fine and dandy — you have to. You can't let yourself down without a fight, you know, and even when you realize that you're on the losing end, you still have to fight. You don't want to be caught dueling there, and just because of a moment's disattention, you get your head cut off. You continue the duel and say, "Hey, if

you're going to get me, buddy [death], you'll have to get me, but I'm going to make you sweat for it.''

Conclusion

The patients' main resource came from within themselves; the spouses relied more on outside support. External resources for the patients came mostly from spouses; spouses' external resources came from family and friends. Generally, it was enough for the patients to be with their spouses. The spouses, however, expressed more need for contact with others and to be more active socially. Two groups of patients were identified according to their perceptions of the nearness of their death; patients perceived their death as uncertain or as inevitable. Both patients and spouses engaged in work which allowed them to manage the diagnosis of advanced cancer. Each type of work for both patients and spouses had a goal and a focus and required the utilization of energy and resources for the goals to be accomplished. The focus and progression toward meeting the goals were different for both patients and spouses depending on to which group the patient belonged. Spouses however described more uncertainty, even when the patient was able to describe the inevitable outcome.

DISCUSSION

The results of this study support a broad view of the concept of work which includes various types of work applied toward dealing with advanced cancer in the family. Work, as it is described in this investigation, provides the context for behaviors used by patients and spouses as they manage advanced cancer at home.

The concept of work has been applied to the adjustment of family members following the death of a loved one. Lindemann (1944) in his classic description of grief responses, used the term "grief work" to encompass the behavior used to separate from the deceased and to readjust to life without a loved one. If it is appropriate to think of an individual engaging in work after the death of a loved one, then it would also seem appropriate to think of family members, and the patient, engaging in work prior to the loss as well.

The concept of work as applicable to illness management is supported by other literature. One of the first references to patient work was identified by Janis (1958) who described "worry work" as the anticipatory process of patients preparing themselves for surgery. Similarly, in this study, there was an element of worry work in the preparing work of patients. Patients worried about how to prepare their families for the uncertain or inevitable outcome of death. The specific work of hospitalized patients has been noted (Corbin & Strauss, 1988; Fagerhaugh, Strauss, Suczek, & Wiener, 1987; Stepter, 1981; Strauss, Fagerhaugh, Suczek, & Wiener, 1981). One similarity between these reports and the current findings relates to the description (Strauss et al., 1981) of patients' "body work" as expenditure of energy and time, accompanied by the courage and will to maintain composure. In the present study, the effort of daily living work for patients involved using energy, with courage and will, to attempt to live as normal a life as possible while at home.

The findings of this study are further supported by Corbin and Strauss (1988) in their detailed description of the concept of work within the context of chronic illness management. They identified three main types of work: everyday work, illness work, and biographical work. Everyday work included those tasks necessary to keeping a job and caring for a home. Spouses in this study also described such work, categorized as surviving work. Instead of being taxed by the demands of this work however, spouses described the vital role of these tasks in providing a diversion. For patients, every day work was categorized as daily living work and involved those tasks which permitted patients to live as normal a life as possible. Although requiring energy and resources, the surviving work of spouses and the daily living work of patients also provided a way of managing the emotional strain of facing an uncertain or inevitable future.

Similarities also exist between Corbin and Strauss' (1988) category of illness work and the category of helping work identified for spouses in this study. Through their helping work, which was directed toward providing for the patients' physical and emotional comfort, spouses engaged in illness work. For patients in this study, illness work was in the background, or foreground, of nearly all their work. One specific type of patient work in this study related to illness work, but not identified as such by Corbin and Strauss, was fighting work.

Parallels between biographical work and the work of patients and spouses in this study can also be drawn in relation to maintaining and preserving work. In all these categories, there is a focus on coming to terms with the illness, adjusting to changed function, and restructuring a view of self. Finally, Corbin and Strauss identified a change in focus depending on the stage of patient illness. In this study also, patients' work had a different focus depending on whether death was perceived as uncertain or inevitable.

Although relatively little has been written about patient work, even less has been published about the possibility that spouses engage in work when their husbands or wives are seriously ill. Fagerhaugh et al. (1987) mentioned that families have safety work to do when a loved one is hospitalized; they imply, however, that the work is the same for both patients and families. The results of this current study show that although some of the patient and spouse work requires similar behaviors, only one area of work is the same for both patients and spouses. Family focused care often implies that health professionals must view the family, or any subsystem thereof, as a unit. In principle, this is correct. However, one cannot view the unit as a whole without giving consideration to the individuals who make up the unit. The results of this study enhance our understanding of the behavior, the "work," of each member of the marital subsystem, of the "fit" between them, and of the contribution of each to the home management of advanced cancer in one member.

IMPLICATIONS FOR PRACTICE AND RESEARCH

The results of this study have the limitations inherent in the qualitative grounded theory method. The use of a small sample and emphasis upon depth rather than breadth of information means that the generalizability of the findings can be established only by further study and comparison with other subject groups. Furthermore, since all participants were Caucasian, the results may not hold true for couples of other cultural backgrounds. At the same time however, the results may enhance understanding of the experience of patients and spouses who are facing the final stages of a life-threatening illness. The findings also have utility in the directions they suggest for further research and practical interventions in the area.

Practice

The notion of patients and spouses as workers removes any sense that they are passive recipients of professional health care services. Hopefully this fact may assist to change any reluctance on the part of health care professionals to share information with patients and spouses. Patients and spouses in this study wanted information on the disease, its prognosis, and treatment. In addition, they wanted this information given in understandable terms in a compassionate manner.

Providing emotional support to patients and families presents a constant challenge for health care professionals. Nurses, for example, are consistently referred to as providers of emotional support; however, what that means is rarely addressed. The notion that patients' and spouses' work may help to identify methods of helping. For example, knowing that spouses need to review their lives with the patient and to discuss their husband's and wife's character, can reassure health professionals that listening to these life reviews is one method of providing emotional support. Results also indicate that patients need to discuss the seriousness of their illness with outsiders, and that health professionals can fulfill this role. Realizing that part of spouses' helping work is to protect the patient can enhance understanding of spouses' protective behaviors and may assist in preventing misunderstanding on the part of hospital staff and families.

Spouses may need assistance in acknowledging that they require diversion from the patient and the illness, especially as the disease progresses. Spouses play a very important role in supporting the patient and carry most of the concern for patients and any children. This makes them a vulnerable group who must be observed for signs of fatigue. Spouses' devotion to their husbands or wives may not allow them to take the time to attend to their own health needs. On the other hand, well-intentioned workers must refrain from taking over too many day-to-day activities of spouses. Such activities assume importance in spouses' survival work.

Research

From the results of this study, work has been identified as an important concept by which to understand the behavior of patients with advanced cancer and their spouse caregivers. Further investigation with larger numbers of individuals in different settings and at different stages of the life cycle is required to validate and further develop the concept of work as it relates to the management of end-stage disease. Questions which remain to be answered are: (a) Do different categories of work occur in families at different points in the life cycle? (b) what is the work of other family members? (c) what is the work of families when a child is the identified patient? (d) how does work differ for families when the patient is hospitalized for palliative care? and (e) how does the work of professional health care workers differ from that of family members?

Designing and carrying out effective supportive programs for families coping with advanced cancer is at present hampered by the lack of adequate research into the coping responses, skills, and difficulties of families in this situation. It is important that future research into this area be built upon a sound basis of qualitative findings, so that our knowledge of the family experience is accurate. Meanwhile, when attempting to facilitate optimal individual and family coping with the end stages of advanced cancer, the importance of understanding the work of patients and spouses cannot be overemphasized.

REFERENCES

Canadian cancer statistics. (1988). Toronto: Canadian Cancer Society.

Cartwright, A., Hockey, L., & Anderson, J.L. (1973). Life before death. Boston: Routledge and Kegan Paul.

Cassileth, B.K., & Hamilton, J.N. (1979). The family with cancer. In B.R. Cassileth (Ed.), The cancer patient (pp. 232-247). Philadelphia: Lea and Bebiger.

Corbin, M.J., & Strauss, A. (1988). Unending work and care: Managing chronic illness at home. San Francisco: Jossey-Bass.

Creek, L.F. (1982). A home care hospice profile: Description, evaluation, and cost analysis. Journal of Family Practice, 14(1), 53-58.

Fagerhaugh, S., Strauss, A.L., Suczek, B., & Wiener, C. (1987). Safety work of patients in the technologized hospital. In K. King (Ed.), *Long term care* (pp. 12-32). New York: Aldine.

Field, P.A., & Morse, J.M. (1985). *Nursing research: The application of qualitative approaches*. London: Croon Helm.

Freihofer, P., & Felton, G. (1976). Nursing behaviors in bereavement: An exploratory study. *Nursing Research, 25*, 332-337.

Glaser, B. (1978). *Theoretical sensitivity*. Mill Valley, CA: Mill Valley Press.

Glaser, B., & Strauss, A. (1967). *The discovery of grounded theory: Strategies for qualitative research*. New York: Aldine.

Gotay, C.C. (1984). *Calgary's palliative home care program: A descriptive study of the second year*. Calgary: Department of Community Health Science, Faculty of Medicine, University of Calgary.

Janis, I.L. (1958). *Psychological stress*. New York: John Wiley & Sons.

LeCompte, M., & Goetz, T.P. (1982). Problems of reliability and validity in ethnographic research. *Review of Educational Research, 52*, 31-60.

Lindemann, E. (1944). Symptomatology and management of acute grief. *American Journal of Psychiatry, 101*, 141-148.

Martinson, I.M., Moldow, O.G., Armstrong, G.D., Henry, W.E., Nesbit, M.E., & Kersey, J.H. (1986). Home care for children dying of cancer. *Research in Nursing and Health, 9*, 11-16.

May, K. (1982). Three phases of father involvement in pregnancy. *Nursing Research, 31*, 331-342.

Mor, D., Greer, D.S., & Kastenbaum, R. (1988). *The hospice experiment*. Baltimore: John Hopkins University Press.

Pringle, D., & Taylor, D. (1984). Palliative care in the home: Does it work? *Canadian Nurse, 80*(6), 26-29.

Stepter, N.G. (1981). Hospitalized patients work. *Supervisor Nurse, 12*(8), 55.

Strauss, A.L., Fagerhaugh, S., Suczek, B., & Wiener, C. (1981). Patients work in the technologized hospital. *Nursing Outlook, 29*, 404-412.

Vachon, M.L.S., Freidman, K., Farmo, A., Rogers, J., Lyall, W.A.L., & Freidman, S.J.J. (1977). The final illness is cancer: The widows perspective. *Canadian Medical Association Journal, 117*, 1151-1154.

Zajac, L.P. (1985). *Review of Edmonton Palliative Home Care*. Edmonton: Home Care Division, Research and Planning Unit.

Social Support:
The Experience
of Hospice Family Caregivers

Jane Marie Kirschling
Virginia Peterson Tilden
Patricia G. Butterfield

SUMMARY. The concepts of social support, reciprocity, cost, and conflict were examined through a methodological study that assessed the reliability and validity of Tilden's (1986) Cost and Reciprocity Index (CRI). The CRI was modified for the face-to-face interviews with 70 family members who were caring for a terminally ill relative enrolled in a hospice program. Item analyses was undertaken with the four subscales because of qualitative comments, a desire to streamline administration of the measure and an overall drop in the alpha coefficients compared with those previously reported. Based on this work 25 items were retained in the four sub-

---

Jane Marie Kirschling, RN, DNS, is Associate Professor of Family Nursing, Oregon Health Sciences University (OHSU), 3181 SW Sam Jackson Park Road, Portland, OR 97201-3098. Virginia Peterson Tilden, RN, DNSc, FAAN, is Professor of Mental Health Nursing at OHSU and is Systemic Family Therapist at the Portland Studies Institute. During 1986-1989, she was Principal Investigator of a federally funded methodological study of the development of measures for social support. Patricia G. Butterfield, RN, MS, is a doctoral student, School of Nursing, OHSU. Her practice has emphasized home based care in both community health and hospice programs. Prior to her enrollment in the doctoral program, she was employed as Hospice Coordinator at Mountain States Tumor Institute in Boise, ID.

This research was funded by the Center for Nursing Research, Nursing Research Emphasis Grant/Doctoral Programs, 1 R21 NU01489-01, 9/86-9/87. An earlier version of this paper was presented at the 22nd Annual Communicating Nursing Research Conference, Western Institute of Nursing, San Diego, CA, May, 1989. The first author wishes to acknowledge the contributions of the graduate research assistants, Georgene Siemsen and James Pittman, to this project.

scales, 13 were eliminated. Cronbach's alpha coefficients and the average inter-item correlation for the revised subscales are reported. Correlation analysis of the revised subscales was also undertaken in order to explore the relationship among the subscales and with time since the care receiver's diagnosis.

A 78 year old woman caring for her 79 year old husband: The only thing I'm worry about is my two daughters—they don't come around to say hi mom, you're doing a good job. I need encouragement. I'm sure they feel I'm doing the best I can . . . I call my son or daughter-in-law because they come willingly. If it came down to the wire the girls would come. They don't offer, don't seem to want to be around him. I think it hurts them, they love him. He's been our rock.

A 38 year old man caring for his 72 year old mother: I have a brother who's an alcoholic, but doesn't admit it. There needs to be frequent reminders for him to make contacts with her and share duties.

A 62 year old woman caring for her 67 year old husband: I've been very reluctant to (ask family for help), but when push came to shove I did and they were right here. Even got a call from daughter-in-law saying whenever we need our son to call. Older daughter lives with us, she is working and going to school. One of the things that clinched her decision to move in was to help, and she does.

Research over the past 20 years has consistently demonstrated what many family members already know; that the family is the primary source of support for older adults (Rabin & Stockton, 1987). In addition to family support, the need for some form of home care increases as family members advance in age. Because of the complex needs of the terminally ill, home hospice care often reflects an intensive level of home-based services. Like home care, the potential need for hospice services increases with advanced age. The physical and emotional needs of the terminally ill mandate an efficient mobilization of both family and professional resources. As home-based services increase, usually so does the involvement of the family in the coordination and provision of care.

The health care system assumes that the family will rally to the challenge of caring for an ill member in the home, yet many health care professionals often have an inadequate understanding of the physical and psychological effects of caregiving on family members. An understanding of the dynamics of support networks is essential for nurses and other health professionals who want to achieve a harmonious coordination of home-based care.

The opening vignettes are taken from interviews with family members of hospice patients. As they illustrate, support from family and friends is critical to the ability of caregivers to manage during this time of crisis. The purpose of this article is to describe selected findings from a study of family members caring for a terminally ill relative using a measure of social support and social network. The concept of social support is discussed, followed by a description of the measure and results related to the measure, and discussion of the findings as they relate to the clinical practice of hospice care providers.

SOCIAL SUPPORT

The support of the social environment has been demonstrated to have a profound effect on health promotion and restoration (for review of the vast research see Broadhead et al., 1983). Cumulative research findings indicate that social support can aid in recovery from hospitalization, surgery, and illness; reduce pregnancy complications for women under high stress; protect against psychological distress in adverse situations; and mediate some of the stress of maturational processes (Hamburg & Killilea, 1979).

Although the definitions of social support vary in the scientific literature, House (1981) noted similar components: emotional support refers to trust, caring, and intimacy; appraisal support refers to feedback that affirms one's self-worth; informational support consists of useful advice and information; and instrumental support refers to tangible goods and services. Definitions of social support have emphasized positive dimensions (Tilden, 1985). This has occurred despite acknowledgement by many writers that social interactions are neither free, nor always benevolent. Wellman (1981) said that not all ties are necessarily supportive and urged the use of the term "social network" in order to avoid the positive bias implied in the term "social support." House also made reference to the costs of maintaining relationships in the reciprocal exchange of time, energy, goods, and services. Kahn and Antonucci (1980) said that if a person sees him- or herself as receiving more support than deserved or can be repaid, the benefits of the support may be dampened. Schaefer, Coyne and Lazarus (1981), and later Broadhead et al. (1983), commented that social relationships are sources of stress as well as support. Indeed, a significant share of stresses people experience in their daily lives emanate from interpersonal relationships.

Instruments that measure social support have perpetuated the bias by taping primarily positive subdimensions. For example, Brandt and Weinert's (1981) PRQ measures nurturance, intimacy, worth, guidance, and social integration. The Norbeck Social Support Questionnaire (Norbeck, Lindsey, & Carrieri, 1981) measures aid, affect, and affirmation. Eckenrode and Gore (1981) said that a major methodological flaw of measurement to date has been the treatment of stress and social support as separate and independent variables. Just as in the recent past, stress was viewed as acontextual and often measured simply as units of change, so support is measured currently as separate from stress. The assumptions here are, first, that sources of support differ from sources of stress, and second, that support systems do not relate causally to stress occurrences. Clearly, both assumptions are violated for most people on a day-to-day basis.

Both the social networks that provide support and the quality of support they provide are affected by terminal illnesses. The dying family member may be unable to reciprocate support received, which places a strain on the network. The family caregiver is faced with the burden of caring for the terminally ill person which can tax the immediate family members emotionally, physically, and financially.

There is initial evidence that an intensive commitment to home care of a terminally ill person by a family member over a protracted period has a negative effect on the caregiver's ability to readjust during the early months after the death (Mor, Greer, & Kastenbaum, 1988). Deterioration in the health status of family members and the family caregiver who have experienced the emotional effects of the death of a terminally ill person can occur during their grieving. The social network of the surviving family members changes with the death of the terminally ill person. In addition there may be the additional loss of friends whose primary relationship was with the deceased.

Social support, reciprocity, cost, and conflict are relevant concepts when considering the experiences of family members who are caring for a terminally ill relative enrolled in a hospice program. Given the positive and negative aspects of social network, it is essential that researchers have a reliable and valid measure that taps these multiple dimensions of social networks.

DESCRIPTION OF RESEARCH

This research was part of a larger methodological study designed to assess the reliability and validity of selected measures. The measures evaluated in the larger study included: Tilden's (1986) Cost and Reciprocity Index, Archbold and Stewart's (1984) caregiving measures, Jalowiec's (1979) Jalowiec Coping Scale, and Paloutzian and Ellison's (1982) Spiritual Well-being Scale. Only findings related to the Cost and Reciprocity Index are described in this article. For those interested, findings for the Spiritual Well-being Scale are described elsewhere (Kirschling & Pittman, 1989).

Cost and Reciprocity Index

The Cost and Reciprocity Index (CRI), developed by the second author, is a self-report questionnaire that taps both structure and function of social networks and yields scores for social support, reciprocity, cost, and conflict. Impetus to develop the instrument came from the desire to correct the biases of existing measures toward only positive dimensions of social networks. The CRI has evolved in form and focus through successive phases of testing (see note 1), from which indices of reliability and validity have been reported (Tilden & Galyen, 1987; Tilden & Nelson, 1988; Tilden & Stewart, 1985).

Conceptual framework. Conceptually, the CRI is based on social exchange theory and equity theory. Social exchange and equity theories contain propositions that help explain the stress-producing aspects of interpersonal relationships. Social exchange theory (Blau, 1964; Cook, 1987; Homans, 1974) holds that human behavior can be explained in terms of rewards that satisfy a person's needs. People attempt to maximize rewards and minimize losses; in order to induce rewards from another person, one must provide rewards in return. Thus, social behavior is an exchange of mutually rewarding activities in which the receipt of rewards is contingent on the supply of benefits returned. People join together insofar as it is in their mutual interest to do so. Therefore, social support is neither "free" nor undirectional.

Equity theory (Burgess & Huston, 1979; Foa, 1971; Messick & Cook, 1983) involves perceptions of justice. According to equity theory, people perceive a balance between costs (investments or expenditures) and rewards (return on investments). An imbalance of exchange can be tolerated for different reasons and periods of time, but generally speaking, stress results when actors see their relationship as unequal or nonreciprocal. The overbenefited feel guilty because of their favored position, and the underbenefited feel angry because of their smaller return.

Thus, social exchange and equity theories hold that human relationships involve reciprocated exchange of valued commodities, the pursuit of which produces costs and conflicts. Use of these theories suggests that subdimensions of interpersonal relationships within social networks, specifically social support, reciprocity, cost, and conflict, should be measured.

Description of the CRI. Network variables measured with the CRI include size, source, number in household, and proximity of kin. Function of the network is indexed by 38 Likert-type items in four subscales. The subscales consist of: (a) *social support* (10 items), defined as perceived enactment or availability of emotional, appraisal, informational, and instrumental supplies, the four components of social support designed by House (1981); (b) *reciprocity* (9 items), defined as perceived equity or balance in relationships, and the extent to which the subject returns as well as receives support; (c) *cost* (6 items), defined as perceived effort and output expended to others in order to maintain relationships; and (d) *conflict* (13 items), defined as perceived tension, disaccord, or stress resulting from relationship within the network. Item responses can range from "not at all" (0), to a "great deal" (4) on a five point scale. Sample items for the four subscales of the CRI are provided in Table 1.

The CRI involves three steps. First, subjects identify the people who are important to them and their relationship with the identified persons. Next, subjects are asked to identify the five most important people, referred to as the inner network throughout the remainder of this article. In the third step the subject responds to 38 questions for each person listed in the inner network.

Psychometric properties of the CRI were evaluated in a sample of 43 patients who were participants in a health maintenance organization obesity program and 218 undergraduate college students

Table 1

Sample Items for the CRI Subscales: Social Support, Cost, Reciprocity and
Conflict

SOCIAL SUPPORT

How much can you count on these people to be there for you no matter what happen?
How often do you learn useful ideas or information from these people?

COST

How much time do you put into these relationships?
How much effort do you put into these relationships?

RECIPROCITY

How often do these people come to you for advice and information?
How often do these people come to you for a boost in spirits?

CONFLICT

How much trouble for any reason are these people to you?
How much unhelpful or unwelcome advice do you get from these people?

(Tilden & Nelson, 1988). Reliability (internal consistency, and test-retest stability) and construct validity were assessed. Internal consistency for the total sample (N = 261) as assessed by Cronbach's alpha was high for all subscales (social support .92; reciprocity .86; cost .89; conflict .94). Test-retest reliability was assessed on a subsample (N = 36) using a two week interval. All scales were reasonably stable (social support r = .90; reciprocity r = .76; cost r = .84; conflict r = .86). Intercorrelations of subscales indicated that social support correlated moderately with other subscales and in expected directions (reciprocity r = .55; cost r = .47; and conflict r = −.23).

Social desirability response set bias was assessed by correlating the subscales with data form the short form of the Marlow-Crowne Social Desirability Index (Strahan & Gerbasi, 1972). Near zero correlations were found for social support, cost, and conflict. Reciprocity correlated weakly (.23), which may be understood in light of people's unconscious need to inflate how much they do for others.

A preliminary factor analysis (N = 261) revealed a strong 3-factor solution (support, reciprocity, and conflict), and did not show cost to be a strong subscale. Some cost items tended to load on each of the three primary factors. Because this was preliminary analysis with a relatively small sample, and because the cost items are indicated by the conceptual framework, they were retained in the CRI.

Revisions in the CRI. The CRI was originally designed for self-administration. In the present study, the research team decided to conduct face-to-face interviews in order to maximize the likelihood of having complete data for the majority of subjects due to the large number of measures and complexity of some of the measures. Therefore, interviewers administered the CRI and recorded responses.

Pilot testing of the CRI indicated that several modifications were necessary to enhance its validity with a caregiver sample. First, subjects were allowed to list an unlimited number of individuals in their social network. Second, subjects were asked to think of the persons they listed as part of their inner network as a group and answer the 38 questions for the group as a whole. With the original

CRI the subjects would have been asked to answer the questions for each individual listed in the inner network. In addition, if caregivers listed the care receiver as a part of their larger network then they were instructed *not* to include the care receiver as one of the members of their inner network. The rationale for this change was that the intent was to use the CRI in a longitudinal study of family caregivers both prior to and after the death of their terminally ill older family member. Consequently, the inclusion of the care receiver in the inner circle would have automatically influenced the composition of the post-death inner circle since he/she would no longer be listed due to death.

Method

During 1986 and 1987 five hospice programs in two northwestern states participated in the study. During a six-month period 63% of the caregivers referred to the study agreed to participate. The criteria for participation were that the care receiver was at least 40 years of age and had been admitted to the hospice program for at least two weeks. Caregivers were sent a letter describing the research and were contacted by phone to determine their willingness to participate. If the caregiver agreed, a time and place for the interview was established.

After the consent form was signed the trained interviewer administered the interview guide and recorded the responses. The interviewer recorded all of the subject's responses during the interview and made notes in the comments section of the guide when he or she elaborated on a specific question.

Sample

The sample of 70 caregivers included 51 women and 19 men who were caring for a terminally ill relative receiving hospice services at home. Caregivers ranged in age from 27 to 84 years, with a mean age of 62.3. The majority of subjects were caring for their spouses (68.6%). The care receivers ranged in age from 48 to 86 years, with a mean age of 71.2. The care receivers had been enrolled in hospice an average of 64.1 days and the time since diagnosis ranged from 1 to 312 months, with a mean time of 33 months. For additional information on the sample the reader is referred to Kirschling and Pittman (1989).

RESULTS

The number of persons identified as part of the caregiver's social network ranged from 4 to 150, with a mean of 17.4 persons. The overwhelming majority of caregivers (99%) identified the care receiver as part of their larger social network. The mean number of persons identified as being most important, or part of the inner network, was 5.3 (range 1 to 18). Children (83%), other relatives (43%), friends (39%), and siblings (33%) were most often included as part of the inner network.

Cronbach's alpha coefficients were calculated on the 38 items which tap four subscales of the CRI. The findings for the 70 caregivers, as well as previously reported results for 218 college students and 43 health care consumers (Tilden, 1987), are provided in Table 2. Overall, alpha coefficients for the hospice family caregivers were lower than from subjects in Tilden's study. A few caregivers had difficulties understanding some of the items or were reluctant to share this type of information with the interviewer. For example, the item "How much do these people care about you, that is like or love you?" elicited the following comments "I haven't thought about it" and "Who thought of this, I'm not a mind reader." Another item that read "How much money do you spend on these people?" elicited a variety of comments including "I'm not going to tell you," "None to spend," "my wife spends money, I don't," and "More than most, what do you mean?" .

Item analyses were undertaken with the four subscales because of the lower alpha coefficients, the qualitative comments, and the first author's desire to streamline administration of the measure. Based on this work 25 items were retained in the four subscales, 13 were eliminated. The decision to retain an item in the subscale was based on its contribution to the reliability of the scale and the type and number of comments caregivers had made about the item. Reliability information on the revised subscales is provided in Table 2.

Mean scores, standard deviations and ranges for the revised subscales are provided in Table 3. Standard means for the subscales

Table 2

CRI: Internal Consistency Reliability Information

| | Original Subscales | | | | | | Revised Subscales | | |
| | Hospice Caregivers | | | Tilden's Sample | | | Hospice Caregivers | | |
	Cron. Alpha	Inter-Item Corr.	n	Cron. Alpha	Inter-Item Corr.		Cron. Alpha	Inter-Item Corr.	n
Support	.80	.27	69	.92	.19		.79	.35	69
Cost	.55	.17	69	.89	.21		.68	.36	70
Reciprocity	.73	.23	67	.86	.12		.82	.43	67
Conflict	.76	.26	68	.94	.19		.83	.41	68

85

Table 3

Hospice Caregivers: Revised CRI Subscales

Subscale	# Items	Mean	sd	Range	n	Stand. Mean	sd
Support	7	17.99	4.89	3-28	69	2.57	.70
Cost	4	10.56	2.63	5-16	70	2.64	.66
Reciprocity	6	12.40	4.36	3-22	67	2.07	.73
Conflict	8	2.91	3.43	0-20	68	.36	.43

Scoring: 0 = Never, none, not at all; 1 = A little, occasionally,
          2 = A moderate amount; 3 = Quite a bit; 4 = A great deal

(mean divided by the number of items in the subscales) are also provided in Table 3. The caregiver reported experiencing a moderate amount of cost ($M = 2.64$), support ($M = 2.57$), and reciprocity ($M = 2.07$) with their inner network; they reported very little ($M = .36$) conflict with their inner network. Tilden's sample of college students and health care consumers also experienced a moderate amount of cost ($M = 2.53$), support ($M = 2.83$), and reciprocity ($M = 2.24$). However, the college students and health care consumers reported greater conflict ($M = .13$) than the hospice caregiver sample.

Correlation analysis of the four revised subscales was undertaken in order to explore the relationship among the subscales. Table 4 includes information on Tilden's (1987) sample of college students and health care consumers and the hospice caregivers.

The correlation coefficients for the two samples are relatively similar and the relationships among the subscales are consistent with the theoretical underpinnings of the CRI. For both samples, support was highly related to reciprocity (.55 and .69), and reciprocity was highly related to cost (.62). Support and conflict were inversely correlated but low. Reciprocity and cost had very little relationship with conflict.

Finally, correlation analysis was undertaken to explore the relationship between time since the care receiver's diagnosis and the

Table 4

Correlation Analysis of CRI Subscales

	Tilden's (1987) Correlation Analysis of Subscales			
	Support	Reciprocity	Cost	Conflict
Support		.55	.47	-.23
Reciprocity			.62	-.02
Cost				-.05

	Hospice Caregivers Correlation Analysis of Revised Subscales			
	Support	Reciprocity	Cost	Conflict
Support		.69	.30	-.18
Reciprocity			.62	.07
Cost				.22

four subscales. Time since diagnosis and cost, reciprocity and support were inversely correlated ($-.10$, $-.20$, and $-.22$ respectively), but low. Time since diagnosis and conflict were not correlated (.02).

DISCUSSION AND CLINICAL IMPLICATIONS

The social support of family members caring for a terminally ill older person enrolled in a hospice program was explored using the Cost and Reciprocity Index (CRI). Issues of reliability and validity of the CRI were explored and the measure was modified in order to streamline administration of the measure and increase the reliability of the four subscales.

A common problem in gerontological research is the wording of items and the overall applicability of the statement to an older person. This most often occurs when the content domain for the instrument was tapped from younger informants, resulting in item syntax that is not familiar to many older persons. Some examples, based on comments made by subjects in the current study, illustrate this issue. Caregivers were asked to identify the people who are important to them. One caregiver responded "there are so many friends, church and family — they're not all close but they are caring . . . the number of closest friends, truly concerned, couldn't begin to list." Another caregiver explained "there are so many people I don't know how to pick them out . . . I don't see them very often (grandchildren) . . . sometimes you know someone really well but their name escapes you." Although there is not a simple solution to the issue of the wording of items in measures developed with younger samples and overall applicability of items for older persons, the issue does underscore the need to continually evaluate the reliability and validity of a measure when the measure is being used with a new population.

The negative dimensions of social support, cost and conflict, appear to be relevant concepts clinically for family members who are caring for a terminally ill relative, despite lower alpha coefficients for these subscales and the relatively low level of conflict in this sample. The reliability and validity information provided in this article do provide initial support for the use of the CRI with hospice family caregivers.

The lower alpha coefficients for the original subscales reported in Table 2 might be due to a variety of reasons, including the changes made in the instrument and the older age of the subjects compared to Tilden's sample. As discussed previously, the lower alpha coefficient for cost may reflect that the measure takes on a different meaning when a caregiver is confronted with issues related to the eventual death of a family member. Also, the psychometric issue of social desirability cannot be dismissed with this sample. During the provision of care for a loved one, hospice caregivers may feel especially vulnerable and be reluctant to acknowledge conflict in their network or risk being perceived as "ungrateful."

A related hypothesis is that caregivers may need to deny or minimize issues of cost in caring for a dying family member because they are unable to deal with this stressful aspect of their social network. Administration of the CRI at different times during the care receiver's illness would provide an interesting glimpses into the dynamics of caregiver's support network over time. Although the current study was not longitudinal in design it was possible to partially evaluate this hypothesis using Pearson r correlation coefficients. As time since diagnosis increased, the perceived degree of support and reciprocity from the inner network slightly decreased ($r = -.22$ and $-.20$). Cost and conflict were not correlated with time since diagnosis for this sample of caregivers. Consequently, it appears that there may be subtle changes in the positive dimensions of the caregiver's support network. Additional research will be necessary to understand the dynamics of change in one's inner network over time. Ideally, future research efforts can be designed to evaluate changes in the composition of the support network and the positive and negative dimensions of the network for family caregivers over time, with data being collected prior to and after the onset of the illness.

The overall lack of conflict in the caregiver sample is intriguing and deserves further attention. The comments of caregivers about their families at the beginning of the article provide evidence that some caregivers experience conflict with other family members (i.e., the mother's concern over her two daughter's absence from the home and the man's efforts to continually remind his brother to help with their mother's care). Caregivers in an earlier study were also asked about the help that they received from friends and conflict in the friend network was often apparent. The following example illustrates potential conflict:

> *A 72 year old woman caring for her 94 year old father*: Friends will come visit but don't want to be responsible. . . . My parents have all these friends—I thought I could go to the stores for 1/2 hour, well forget it. Several say if you have to have me, call me, but they are busy when I call. Lots of friends come and see them and bring them goodies—but when it comes to nitty-gritty—don't think so.

Since these comments came from caregivers who participated in another study it was impossible to verify whether the caregivers identified the relatives and friends that they talked about within their inner networks. Although speculative, it appears that at least in the case of the mother she would have included the daughters in her inner network. It is less clear whether the daughter would have included her friends, and her parent's friends, as part of her inner network.

The overall low level of conflict in the caregiver's inner network may reflect the caregiver's unwillingness to acknowledge conflict or share this information with the interviewer. Tilden, Nelson, and May (in press) also found low levels of conflict in a sample of persons with cancer, as compared with samples of community residents, thus illustrating the hypothesis that people in situations of terminal illness either do not experience or do not acknowledge interpersonal conflict. The finding may be explained, in part, by the line of reasoning that when older persons find themselves in a situation where there is a great deal of conflict they may decide to exclude the person(s) from their inner network.

Clinical Implications

Although the purpose of this methodological study was to evaluate the reliability and validity of an existing measure of social support with a sample of hospice caregivers, the results highlight some issues that hospice clinicians may want to consider. First, social support includes both positive and negative aspects. As hospice team members interact with the caregiver, they should explore the support available to the caregiver in relation to cost, reciprocity and conflict. For example, a caregiving wife may have adult children in the area who could be called upon to help out; however if she perceives that the cost would be too great or that she experiences a great deal of conflict with a specific child, she may be unwilling to mobilize this support.

Hospice clinicians will, on occasion, interface with a family caregiver who identifies a great deal of conflict in his or her relationships. When this situation presents itself it may be useful to explore with the caregiver how these individuals fit into their inner support network. In the situation where the conflicted relationship is a central one, then the clinician may decide to intervene in order to resolve the conflict. This may include making a referral to a mental health specialist. If the relationship is not central, then the clinician may choose to refocus the conversation toward relationships that are perceived as more important.

A second issue involves the variability among caregivers in terms of the size of their social network and inner network. The social networks ranged from 4 to 150 people and the inner network ranged any where from 1 to 18 people. The authors would caution clinicians against viewing bigger as better. The degree of support that an individual receives needs to be evaluated in terms of the caregiver's perception of whether he or she feels supported, and whether the relationships are reciprocal, the costs are within reason, and the level of conflict is tolerable.

Finally, hospice clinicians need to work with the caregiver and the terminally ill person within the context of their support networks. This may include allowing the caregiver to ventilate his or her frustration over the lack of friends who visit the dying person family member, offering to teach friends or family members how to care for the ill persons while the caregiver goes to the store, or arranging a family meeting in order to work through issues about caring for the terminally ill family member.

Hospice team members provide formal support to families during the stressful time when a member is dying. As families become comfortable with the hospice staff it is not unusual for them to begin to perceive the staff as part of the family. Because of the closeness that often develops between staff and family during the intensity of the death experience, hospice providers may need to remind themselves that their supportive functions are within the professional, rather than the family domain (Kirschling, 1988). The caregiver's naturally occurring support network should not be forgotten or ignored, but should be enhanced through effective coordination of care. The caregiver's long standing relationships with family and friends will provide the foundation for social support in the months and years following the death of the terminally ill family member.

NOTE

1. The final form of the measure, called the Interpersonal Relationship Index (IPRI), has undergone extensive psychometric evaluation and is currently in widespread use by investigators. The IPRI is a 39-item measure of social support, reciprocity, and conflict, and in addition is available in a 26-item short form. Copies may be obtained by writing the second author at the Oregon Health Sciences University, Department of Mental Health Nursing, EJSN, 3181 SW Sam Jackson Park Road, Portland, OR 97201-3098.

REFERENCES

Archbold, P.G., & Stewart, B. (1984). *The effects of organized family caregiver relief*. Division of Nursing Research Grant. The Oregon Health Sciences University School of Nursing, Portland, OR.

Blau, P. (1964). *Exchange and power in social life*. New York: Wiley.

Brandt, P., & Weinert, C. (1981). The PRQ — a social support measures. *Nursing Research, 30*, 277-280.

Broadhead, W.E., James, S.A., Wagner, E.H., Schoenback, V.J., Grimson, R., Heyden, S., Tibblin, G., & Gehlbach, S. (1983). The epidemiologic evidence for a relationship between social support and health. *American Journal of Epidemiology, 117*, 521-537.

Burgess, R.L., & Huston, T.L. (1979). *Social exchange in developing relationships*. New York: Academic Press.

Cook, K.S. (1987). *Social exchange theory*. Beverly Hills, CA: Sage

Eckenrode, E.S., & Gore, S. (1981). Stressful events and social supports: The significance of context. In B.H. Gottlieb (Ed.), *Social networks and social support* (pp. 43-68). Beverly Hills, CA: Sage.

Foa, U.G. (1971). Interpersonal and economic resources. *Sciences, 171*, 345-351.

Hamburg, D.A., & Killilea, M. (1979). Relation of social support, stress, illness, and use of health services. In *Healthy people: The Surgeon General's report on health* (pp. 253-276). Washington, D.C.: U.S. Government Printing Office.

Homans, G.C. (1974). *Social behavior: Its elementary forms* (revised ed.). New York: Harcourt.

House, J.S. (1981). *Work stress and social support*. Reading, MA: Addison-Wesley.

Jalowiec, A. (1979). *Jalowiec Coping Scale*. University of Illinois, Chicago, IL.

Kahn, R.L., & Antonucci, T.C. (1980). Convoys over the life course: Attachment roles, and social support. In P.B. Batles & O.G. Brim (Eds.), *Life-span development and behavior* (Vol 3) (pp. 254-286). New York: Academic Press.

Kirschling, J.M. (1988). Hospice care for aging families: An opportunity to promote family well-being. In L. Krentz (Ed.), *Workshop Proceedings: Nursing and the Promotion/Protection of Family Health* (pp. 117-142). Portland, OR: Oregon Health Sciences University, Department of Family Nursing.

Kirschling, J.M., & Pittman, J.F. (1989). Measurement of spiritual well-being: A hospice caregiver sample. *The Hospice Journal, 5*(2), 1-11.

Messick, D.M., & Cook, K.S. (1983). *Equity theory*. New York: Praeger.

Mor, V., Greer, D.S., & Kastenbaum, R. (1988). *The hospice experiment*. Baltimore: The John Hopkins University Press.

Norbeck, J.S., Lindsey, A.M., Carrieri, V.L. (1981). The development of an instrument to measure social support. *Nursing Research, 30*, 264-269.

Paloutzian, R.F., & Ellison, C.W. (1982). Loneliness, spiritual well-being and the quality of life. In L.A. Peplau & D. Perlman (Eds.), *Loneliness a source-*

book of current theory, research and therapy (pp. 224-237). New York: John Wiley & Sons.

Rabin, D.L., & Stockton, P. (1987). *Long-term care for the elderly a factbook*. New York: Oxford University Press.

Schaefer, C., Coyne, J.C., & Lazarus, R.S. (1981). The health-related functions of social support. *Journal of Behavioral Medicine, 4*, 381-406.

Strahan, R., & Gerbasi, K.C. (1972). Short, homogenous versions of the Marlow-Crowne Social Desirability Scale. *Journal of Clinical Psychology, 28*(2), 191-193.

Tilden, V.P. (1986). *CRI*. Oregon Health Sciences University, Portland, OR.

Tilden, V.P. (1985). Issues of conceptualization and measurement of social support in the construction of nursing theory. *Research in Nursing and Health, 8*, 199-206.

Tilden, V.P. (1987). Summary of the CRI pilot testing. *Report on BRSG project*. Oregon Health Sciences University.

Tilden, V.P., & Galyen, R.D. (1987). Cost and conflict the darker side of social support. *Western Journal of Nursing Research, 9*, 9-18.

Tilden, V.P., & Nelson, C. (1988). Cost and reciprocity index: A measure of interpersonal exchange. Paper presented at the 21st Annual Communicating Nursing Research Conference, WSRN, May 4-6, 1988, Salt Lake City, UT.

Tilden, V.P., Nelson, C., & May, B.A. (in press). The Interpersonal Relationship Inventory: Development and psychometric characteristics. Nursing Research.

Tilden, V.P., & Stewart, B.J. (1985). Problems in measuring reciprocity with difference scores. *Western Journal of Nursing Research, 7*, 381-385.

Wellman, B. (1981). Applying network analysis to the study of support. In B.H. Gottlieb (Ed.), *Social networks and social support* (pp. 171-200). Beverly Hills, CA: Sage.

A Marital Crisis:
For Better or Worse

Jennifer Lillard
Cathy L. McFann

SUMMARY. This case study explores the relationship between Hospice of Marin's initial psychosocial assessment and interdisciplinary team communications with overall treatment outcomes. A brief review of literature is followed by presentation of methods and results. A final critical discussion suggests directions for further research.

REVIEW OF LITERATURE

This report of hospice involvement in a family crisis is based on the case study method of research. Although sometimes viewed skeptically, this approach is clearly a valid investigative structure within accepted parameters. Essentially, it is an extensive examination of a single subject or unit of analysis. One or more situations in which the unit occurs are explored over time using a variety of data collection tools. The case study may be particularly appropriate

Jennifer Lillard, RN, MS, is Nurse Team Coordinator at Hospice of Marin and Assistant Clinical Professor at the University of California San Francisco School of Nursing. She has been involved in hospice work since 1976, is a member of the National Hospice Organization, the Oncology Nursing Society, and Sigma Theta Tau. Cathy L. McFann, MFCC, ADTR, MA, is Social Services Coordinator at Hospice of Marin, is in private practice as Marriage and Family Counselor, and is a consultant to Medical Ergonomic Therapeutic Services. She has been involved in hospice work since 1987 and is a member of the California Association of Marriage and Family Counselors.

The authors gratefully acknowledge contributions made by Tish Bulkley, M.Div.; Cathy Butler, RN; Nancy Langley, MSW; Linda Silver, RN, MFCC, MA; Janet Winegarner, RN; and Michael F. Hoyt, PhD.

when the relationship between the involved variables is complex and somewhat unclear (Polit & Hungler, 1986). It is often used in the early stage of a research investigation to generate hypotheses needing further study and is especially attractive in situations where qualitative aspects are more important than quantitative ones (Woods & Mitchell, 1988). The format is less restricted by established procedures than other study approaches (Meier & Pugh, 1986). Commonly, results are generalized from a single case to one or more subsequent cases and are further examined using another research design.

Also especially relevant to this study is the literature related to family systems and families in crisis. Since beginning service delivery in 1976, Hospice of Marin (HOM) has considered each patient/family as a complete unit whose major purpose is to promote the well-being of its members. Over time, families develop a homeostasis of relationships and behavioral patterns that are relied upon to satisfy family needs and tasks (Hansen & Hill, 1964).

Family systems show some common characteristics but also have unique developmental and historical experiences which influence them. Thus, all families can be described in terms of their boundaries, cohesion and adaptability although they will vary significantly within each of these dimensions (Minuchin & Fishman, 1981). If life events disrupt the usual homeostasis or pattern of coping, all the members of the family group respond in an effort to re-establish a satisfactory balance (Satir, 1968). Depending on a number of factors in the family's history, structure, and functioning, illness and death can have a variable impact on the individual family members and the family organization. Serious end-stage illness and the beginning of hospice service is clearly such a life event and may precipitate a major life crisis accompanied by incapacitating feelings of helplessness, anxiety, massive family disruption or over-utilization of established defense patterns (Craig & Abeloff, 1974; Olsen, 1970). Theory and research on the impact of illness trajectories on families suggest that the family unit's response to the crisis directly affects patient outcome as well as the relative success or inadequacy of their long-term adjustment (Bruhn, 1977; Olsen, 1970). Ultimately, the hospice team's goal is to assist the family to effectively manage the unavoidable crisis that death precipitates.

METHODS

HOM is a Medicare-certified home health agency providing service to an average of 33 patients/families at any one time. The average length of stay is 47 days, and during the past year 40% of the patients served have elected the Hospice Medicare Benefit. Marin County, where the agency provides services, is a primarily middle and upper-middle class residential community north of the Golden Gate Bridge from San Francisco.

Care is provided by an interdisciplinary team (IDT) composed of a medical director, nurses, counselors, social workers, home health aides, volunteer coordinator and volunteers, chaplain, liaison nurse and bereavement coordinator. As soon as a referral is received, an informational visit is scheduled with the liaison nurse, and the patient/family is admitted. Each patient/family is followed closely by a primary nurse who is responsible for initial assessment of overall patient/family needs, symptom management, coordination of agency services for the patient/family within the multi-disciplinary team context, ongoing identification of physical problems and prompt readjustment of the plan of care (Lillard & Bystrowski, 1981; Lillard & Marietta, 1989).

Direct psychosocial service includes an initial psychosocial assessment, family and individual counseling, pastoral counseling, a family support group, and ongoing consultation with nursing staff and other involved professionals. A counselor visits shortly after admission to complete a psychosocial assessment (PSA) which identifies family characteristics including communication patterns, roles, immediate problems and coping styles and assists the team in understanding the family, establishing expectations and planning interventions.

IDT communication occurs in both structured and unstructured ways. The full team meets three hours weekly for a comprehensive review of patient/family needs, inter-team communication, consultation, problem solving and treatment planning. Daily reports provide opportunity for ongoing, timely readjustment of plans in response to changing needs and facilitate continual inter-team feedback and support. Patient care staff are seated in close proximity facilitating spontaneous sharing and consultation on an as-needed basis.

The accuracy of the PSA combined with the ongoing effectiveness of IDT care planning communications are significant factors in overall treatment effectiveness. In an effort to further refine the HOM care delivery system, the authors formulated two specific questions: (1) Is the initial PSA format providing adequate, pertinent data? (2) Are ongoing IDT communications complete and consistent? Given the complicated relationship between HOM's PSA and IDT structures to the overall care delivery mission, the case study format is the method of choice at this early stage of exploration.

A patient/family case history was selected for study based on the complexity of the marital relationship, an apparently unpredictable crisis occurring during a home visit by HOM staff, and involvement of a maximum number of team members including nurses, chaplain, and counselor. Although there were adult children in the family constellation, the marital couple's relationship was pivotal and of major concern to the IDT. Consequently the study report focuses on the couple, presenting selected, relevant assessments and interventions that occurred during the course of hospice care. Names and demographics are changed in the report to assure family confidentiality.

The PSA and ongoing IDT communication play particularly crucial roles in this family situation, making this an instructive case study. Two data collection tools were used for the study. Record review included complete evaluation of nursing, chaplain and counseling notes as well as thorough examination of the PSA report. In addition, anecdotal notes of the weekly team meetings and daily reports were studied. The data collection produced a comprehensive, detailed summary of the team's work with the family.

RESULTS

Study results are reported chronologically beginning with the informational visit, followed by three monthly summaries and concluding with the time of death.

Request for Service and Informational Visit

On February 1, 1989, Mary Edwards (a pseudonym) called the Hospice of Marin office following the suggestion of her husband's physician. She said that her husband, Frank, age 70, had prostate cancer and they were both interested in the possibility of assistance from hospice. The liaison nurse immediately phoned the primary physician for clarification of the patient's condition and appropriateness for hospice care and then scheduled an informational visit with the family.

Five days later the liaison nurse met the patient, his wife and their 25-year-old daughter Helen at their home. She explained hospice services, coverage options under Medicare, and gathered some initial information for the hospice database. Mr. and Mrs. Edwards had been married 38 years and had two children — Paul, age 30, and Helen. Paul lived with his wife 25 miles away from his parents' home, and Helen was living independently nearby.

Shortly after their marriage, the Edwards had opened a laundromat that they still operated with a great deal of assistance from their son. Mr. Edwards had been well until three years ago when he was hospitalized for chronic obstructive pulmonary disease (COPD), developed diabetes, and his prostate cancer was simultaneously diagnosed. The cancer had been treated with chemotherapy and hormones, but subsequent metastases to spine, hip, and ribs had resulted in a decision to stop treatment. The couple talked at length about their three-year struggle with chronic illness and expressed some frustration with each other and their need for someone to support them. Mrs. Edwards appeared angry with her husband and requested support from HOM while Helen, the daughter, was generally quiet during the visit.

Admission Visit and Initial Assessments

The following day the primary nurse made an admission visit to the family, obtained signed consents, and completed a physical assessment. At that time, Mr. Edwards needed partial assistance with activities of daily living (ADL's), was constipated, continent, and quite weak, with extra heart sounds, diffuse rales throughout his lungs, and was producing copious amounts of white fluid. He was using oxygen at 1 1/2 liters per minute PRN and complained of pain in his back and mid-chest region. His skin was intact with some ecchymotic areas. He appeared significantly emotionally depressed to the primary nurse but was oriented and lucid.

Daily medications included a long list of cardiac and respiratory agents as well as Oral Morphine Solution (OMS), a stool softener and a bulk laxative. Before leaving the patient's home, the primary nurse phoned the patient's physician to present her assessment and obtained orders to increase the OMS and initiate regular dosing with a therapeutic level of Naprosyn. Upon returning to the office, she charted pain, weakness, respiratory distress, and disturbance of psychosocial functioning on the patient's problem list.

The initial PSA was completed by a counselor soon after the family's admission. The counselor reported little expression of positive feeling between the couple although they spoke of a long marriage and shared commitment to their children. Through the three years of Frank's illness, the couple had made an uneasy transition of roles, with Mary taking over the family business quite confidently. As is often true with families who cope with chronic illness, Frank's prognosis of less than six months was difficult for them to acknowledge. Both expected things to "go on as they have" for an undetermined time.

During the PSA Frank expressed future hopes, a feeling of isolation, and a desire for more support; but he did not appeal directly to Mary for it. The record of the visit states that he was "depressed and discouraged." Mary seemed angry during the interview as she talked about her wish for more distance and time away. Although she intellectually acknowledge her husband's limited prognosis, she remained pragmatically unemotional, expressed commitment to keeping Frank at home and was concerned about the stress of his day-to-day care. The counselor expected that Mary would not be open to direct emotional support but would utilize practical assistance. She also felt that tension and ambivalence was long-standing in the couple's relationship and was intensified by Frank's increasing symptoms and need for care. When the Edwardses' case was discussed for the first time at an IDT meeting, the team decided that Mary should be offered direct counseling and participation in the HOM family support group. She declined both. Frank, however, welcomed the team's suggestion for regular individual counseling, chaplain visits, and supportive visits from a hospice nurse specializing in imagery, relaxation and stress management.

First Month

During the first month of HOM service, the patient and his caregivers presented a number of problems requiring intervention by the primary nurse. Measuring and dispensing medication became an issue, and the nurse spent considerable time reviewing the medications with the couple. She identified the patient's anxiety about the issue, suggested that Mrs. Edwards assume responsibility for the medications, and passed this observation on to the team. Here was early evidence of some ongoing tension between the couple.

Occasionally at daily reports the primary nurse expressed frustration with Mrs. Edwards' absence during home visits and concern for the family's apparent lack of follow-through. The team in general was building a strong allegiance with Frank and finding it difficult to empathize with Mary. Mary appeared irritated when the nurse attempted to explore her feelings about daily care routines and related stress.

Meanwhile, Mr. Edwards developed a stage I decubitus on his coccyx, and difficulty urinating, increased respiratory distress and vomiting although he remained afebrile. The nurse reported the changes to the doctor, initiated Duoderm and an eggcrate mattress, prophylactic antibiotics, Compazine and teaching about related changes in care needs.

About three weeks after beginning hospice service, Mrs. Edwards described feeling increasingly exhausted and overwhelmed with her husband's daily care, so the nurse began home health aide service twice a week. Later in the month, the patient again became constipated, so his dose of stool softeners was raised; Senokot and PRN Dulcolax suppositories were added to his bowel regimen, and the problem resolved. Throughout the month, the nurse continued to identify the patient's emotional depression as a problem and offered active listening in response to his concerns about dying, funeral and memorial preparations.

Unfortunately, due to an illness in her own family, the primary counselor involved with this case was not able to schedule a visit with Mr. Edwards until late in the month. When the counselor did meet with Mr. Edwards, he actively grieved his numerous losses and did some life review to prepare for his death. Meanwhile the chaplain had begun visiting. The primary focus of her visits was spiritual, but many of Frank's anxieties concerning his illness and mortality were also addressed. In team conferences the chaplain shared brief information, but it was not until the retrospective case study review that the significance of the clerical relationship became apparent.

Second Month

During his second month of care, Mr. Edwards experienced some renewed respiratory distress which was relieved with Pulmoiade. His recurrence of constipation necessitated an enema and a review of the established bowel regimen with the patient and his wife. In response to the patient's questions, the primary nurse consulted the physician concerning the patient's disease progression and treatment options. The physician offered a regimen of palliative chemotherapy with less than 50% chance of disease remission, but Mr. and Mrs. Edwards decided not to pursue the option due to the high risk of discomforting side effects. The nurse continued to confer with Mary around practical matters but still found it difficult to engage her around any other issues.

Meanwhile, Mr. Edwards reported that amelioration of his symptoms was allowing him to work on a family photo album that he very much wanted to complete. The nurse encouraged his activity and admired the work as it progressed, providing an opportunity for further life review and reinforcing a quality of life focus. At the end of the month Mr. Edwards developed a viral throat infection which exacerbated his cough, suppressed his appetite and returned his focus to his illness. Although his decubitus had healed, his overall disease progression accompanied by extreme fatigue, marked shortness of breath, and peripheral edema led to two panic episodes during which he had images of choking to death. Not surprisingly, his increase in physical symptoms correlated with a more intense focus on his feelings and anxiety during meetings with the chaplain.

To complicate matters, the primary counselor had a death in her own family and was away during much of this month further delaying her supportive involvement. The IDT decided not to inform the Edwards of the reason for her absence. Other team members — in this case the nurse and chaplain — were asked to address the emerging emotional issues. During continuing visits with the chaplain Frank reviewed his life history, reconciled himself with an estranged friend, explored a number of religious and spiritual themes, and increasingly focused on his concerns and fears about death. He stated that he felt he would never be ready to die. He met with a nurse consultant specializing in imagery and began to use relaxation tapes for stress management.

During the month there were lengthy team discussions about the Edwards' situation. Mrs. Edwards was usually occupied at the laundromat so was not at home during visits by team members. Most nursing contacts with her were by phone. As the patient's symptoms intensified, so did her emotional detachment: the couple's homeostasis was in precarious balance. Despite plans to support the family system as it existed, Frank had established more of an alliance with the hospice team than with his wife and it would be difficult to elicit her involvement.

Recognizing that a couple's session might be demanding and stressful, the team decided to have the chaplain and counselor do a joint visit with the couple's consent, focusing on realistic, practical plans around memorial and funeral decisions rather than directly addressing the emotional issues. However, Mrs. Edwards' level of intensity during the couple's session engendered a question from the chaplain about her emotional state. The counselor's notes of the visit describe Frank as "open, willing to talk, and appropriately tearful." Mary couldn't tolerate the open discussion of feelings and angrily stormed from the room at the point that the chaplain asked her directly about her feelings. There was too much emotional intensity for this couple to tolerate.

Within a day Mr. Edwards presented increased shortness of breath and shortly thereafter he had a sudden onset of sharp pain in his left chest associated with movement. The nurse, after discussing his changed respiratory status with the team, urged him to use Ativan on an around-the-clock basis in conjunction with his other respiratory distress measures. After a thorough nursing assessment of the new pain and consultation with the IDT, the pain was attributed to new bony metastases in the upper rib cage. The patient's morphine dose was increased, pain relief was gradually achieved, and for the next three weeks his symptoms stabilized.

The chaplain and counselor had both felt disturbed by their session with the Edwards, wondering if they had caused pain that might have been avoided. In patient care conference as well as in later meetings together and with supervisors, they spent considerable time analyzing their intervention and the family's response. After review with the IDT, it was agreed that Mary's low tolerance for the expression of feelings and Frank's increased expressiveness were in conflict. It seemed that the explosive expression of emotion may have served the purpose of defusing the increasing level of tension in the couple. Despite the fact that it had been the chaplain who directly questioned Mary on her own emotional status, Mary angrily perceived the counselor as the one who "brought up all that emotional stuff." The team felt that any continued contact by the counselor might be too threatening and suggested the chaplain would continue her visits alone. Mary confirmed this assessment, feeling that the counselor was not acceptable. The exclusion of the counselor may have served symbolically to assist the family in maintaining its sense of integrity and control: the threat was symbolically sent away with the counselor.

Third Month

Fortunately, the chaplain's next visit was a healing one. She began the session with Frank, exploring the difference between a cure and palliative care. Mary joined them at this point, and the three prayed together for some time. Following this, a discussion ensued with both partners sharing the great difficulty of seeing Frank decline and approach death. They had found a safe forum in which to express their pain and tears.

The following visits Frank had with the chaplain focused directly on images of life after death, his grief over his leaving life, and his sadness over the tension between Mary and him. Mary also spoke with the chaplain about her struggles coping with Frank's increased physical symptoms and her uncertainty as to whether she could manage to keep him at home. Frank became distressed and began to speak with the chaplain about his impulses toward suicide. He wanted to "die or get better." His suicidal impulses were at a feeling level, and he expressed no intent to carry them into action. The chaplain was in regular contact with the family throughout the month and consulted regularly with the primary nurse. It was a long and difficult month for the Edwards. Fortunately, Mary had formed enough of an alliance with HOM that she could now reach out for some assistance. She spoke with the chaplain and nurse as Frank's condition declined, receiving confirmation of her own struggle and validation of the difficulty of keeping Frank in the home.

Mr. Edwards' physical condition further deteriorated. He had several episodes of breakthrough pain, engendering increased anger from his wife who resented the unpredictable, PRN dosing and asked for the first time about the possible benefits of convalescent placement. A week later, Frank developed spiking temperatures, marked respiratory secretions and confusion which exacerbated his wife's feelings. In an open statement directly reflecting her ambivalence about the closeness involved in providing his care, Mrs. Edwards told the nurse she didn't think she could continue. The nurse discussed support options with her and encouraged her to use additional back-up from her children. After consultation with the team and physician, Haldol and Scopalamine patches were started to ameliorate the confusion and audible respiratory congestion which were so disturbing to Mrs. Edwards. The patient died three days later at home with his family present and with end-stage symptoms minimized. The primary nurse was called, attended, and found the whole family, particularly Mrs. Edwards, relieved that the long ordeal was over and pleased that Mr. Edwards ultimately had been able to stay at home.

Following Frank's death, the chaplain met with Mary and her children and assisted them in writing a eulogy and planning a memorial service which the chaplain performed. Mary continued to hold her feelings in check after Frank's death, although occasionally she would cry. The final patient care conference reviewed Frank's death and the IDT involvement in the case and provided an opportunity to plan bereavement services. Both Mary and the children were offered individual or group bereavement counseling as well as participation in the bereavement classes and informal socials.

A month later the primary nurse made a bereavement contact and found that Mrs. Edwards was able to sleep well, could talk comfortably about what had happened, was in good physical health, and had returned to work in the family business. She did not utilize any further bereavement services.

DISCUSSION

This research was undertaken to address two important questions: (1) Is the initial psychosocial assessment (PSA) data adequate? and (2) Are on-going interdisciplinary team (IDT) communications complete and adequate? A critical review of results suggests need for improvement in both the PSA and IDT communications. The difficulties confronted by the IDT and the measures taken since conclusion of the study to improve the team's effectiveness are outlined below.

First, in scrutinizing the PSA design and the data obtained, it is clear that some important features of the family system had been identified and utilized in treatment planning. Because of Mr. and Mrs. Edwards' emotional distance, the team decided not to pursue couple's counseling and instead focused on providing each partner with support in ways that were tailored to fit their individual styles. The team was able to build on the long-term commitment between the partners and understood that it was historically focused on the practical issues of running a business and raising children rather than on emotional intimacy such as sharing personal feelings.

However, as Mr. Edwards' disease, dependency and need for emotional expression increased, HOM staff members were frustrated with Mrs. Edwards' response of anger towards him. Without fully understanding the degree to which the family system was closed emotionally distant and threatened by escalating HOM involvement (which paralleled the patient's physical decline), the IDT had not directly cautioned team members, offered needed support for members' feelings, or even anticipated the difficult crisis that resulted in Mrs. Edwards' explosion. The case study indicates that the PSA's design had not satisfactorily outlined the system's relationship to the outside world, (in)flexibility in the face of needed change, or the relative degree of enmeshment. Consequently, the PSA is being revised drawing additional information from Salvador Minuchin's framework describing the continuums of boundaries, cohesion, and adaptability as they present in family systems (Minuchin & Fishman, 1981). It is hoped that additional awareness about these characteristics of family functioning will enable more graceful facilitation of needed family change while supporting functional adaptive styles that exist in family systems.

Second, a review of the patient care communications that occurred during the case also revealed strengths as well as weaknesses. The case was unusual in that the primary counselor was away during the early weeks due to a personal family illness and death. As ideally happens in IDT work, other disciplines — in this situation the nurse and chaplain — were able to provide some interim assessment and support. When the counselor returned and made a joint visit with the chaplain, the couple's stress was certainly intense; but they were still communicating and functioning. However, the chaplain's direct questions about feelings precipitated Mrs. Edwards' angry departure from the meeting. The weakness in IDT communications identified by case review relates to completeness of communication and support when several team members are involved. The chaplain does not attend daily report due to other commitments. While the study was in progress she told the researchers that she is sometimes hesitant to contribute observations or ask for additional information in patient care conference because of perceived time constraints. She felt that more complete discussion of the couple and their needs might have led to a better family conference. As a result of these findings, all IDT members completed a survey questionnaire about their observations, suggestions and concerns related to patient care conference; and changes have been implemented. Specifically, all team members involved in every case discussed are directly asked for comments or questions during the meeting to minimize the risk of inadequate or incomplete discussion.

This case study identified both strengths and weaknesses in the PSA and IDT communications. Changes to improve team effectiveness have been initiated. Both study questions can be further explored in subsequent research: The revised PSA can be evaluated using a single or multiple case study format. In addition, IDT communications should be further examined using a combination of survey and/or case study to explore both formal and informal communication structures used by the IDT. Psychosocial assessment and ongoing interdisciplinary team communication are essential elements in hospice care delivery, and their effectiveness must be maximal in order to best serve patient/families.

This case study also evokes questions about the significance and meaning of crisis for hospice families. As defined in the *Random House Dictionary* (1987), a crisis is "(1) a stage in the sequence of events at which the trend of all future events, especially for better or worse, is determined, and (2) the point in the course of serious disease at which a decisive change occurs leading either to recovery or death." The challenge for hospice staff is not to help families avoid crisis but instead, as the IDT attempted with the Edwardses, to assist them to manage in ways that respect their integrity and facilitate independent decision-making and growth.

REFERENCES

Bruhn, J.G. (1977). Effects of chronic illness on the family. *The Journal of Family Practice, 4*, 1057-1060.

Craig, T., & Abeloff, M. (1974). Psychiatric symptomatology among hospitalized cancer patients. *American Journal of Psychiatry, 131*, 1323-1327.

Hansen, D.A., & Hill, R. (1964). Families under stress. In H.T. Christensen, (Ed.), *Handbook of Marriage and the Family*, (p. 806). Chicago: Rand McNally.

Lillard, J., & Bystrowski, K. (1981). Role strain in hospice nursing. *Home Health Quarterly, 1* (2), 51.

Lillard, J., & Marietta, L. (1989). *Palliative Carl nursing: Promoting family integrity*. In C.L. Gilliss, B.L. Highley, B.M. Roberts, & I.M. Martinson (Eds.), Toward a science of family nursing (pp. 437-460). Menlo Park, CA: Addison-Wesley.

Minuchin, S., & Fishman, H.C. (1981). *Family therapy techniques*. Cambridge, MA: Harvard University Press.

Meier, P., & Pugh, E. J. (1986). The case study approach: A viable approach to clinical research. *Research in Nursing and Health, 9*, 195-202.

Murgatroyd, S., & Woolfe, R. (1985). *Helping families in distress*. London: Harper & Row.

Olsen, E.H. (1970). The impact of serious illness on the family system. *Postgraduate Medicine, 47,* 169-171.

Polit, D. F., & Hungler, B.P. (1987). *Nursing research principles and methods.* (2nd ed.). Philadelphia: J.B. Lippencott.

Random house dictionary. (2nd ed.). (1987). NY: Random House.

Satir, V. (1968). *Conjoint Family Therapy* Palo Alto: Science and Behavior Books.

Silver, L., & Winegarner, J. (1988, November). *Effective reorganization of the hospice interdisciplinary team.* Paper presented at the annual meeting of the National Hospice Organization, Orlando, FL.

Woods, N.F., & Mitchell, P.H. (1988). Designing studies to explore association and differences. In N.F. Woods and M. Catanzaro, *Nursing research,* (pp. 156-163). St. Louis: C.V. Mosby.

For Product Safety Concerns and Information please contact our EU
representative GPSR@taylorandfrancis.com Taylor & Francis Verlag GmbH,
Kaufingerstraße 24, 80331 München, Germany

Printed and bound by CPI Group (UK) Ltd, Croydon, CR0 4YY
08/06/2025
01897007-0001